Contents

Preface

Infections due to two species of hookworm, *Ancylostoma duodenale* and *Necator americanus*, almost ubiquitous over large areas of the tropics and subtropics and of persistently high prevalence, continue to be major causes of iron deficiency anaemia and associated ill-health.

Hookworm infection was the target of major control campaigns from the early years of this century until after the Second World War, yet it stubbornly remains as a marker of deficiencies in sanitation, health education and appreciation of its significance as a public health problem. Lack of interest in control at country level is doubtless a function of the low mortality from hookworm infection combined with the technical difficulties of measuring and quantifying the morbidity directly due to hookworms compared with that due to concomitant complications such as poor nutrition or retarded rates of growth.

In theory, control is simple and attainable through health education from childhood onwards, provision of adequate sanitary facilities, judicious use of the numerous efficient anthelminthics now available and supplementary therapy with iron where necessary.

This manual attempts to redress the somewhat negative image of hookworm as an area unworthy of scientific interest and control effort. Although directed at all categories of health professionals, it is addressed primarily to those practitioners at the peripheral health care level who carry the burden of preventive and curative action, and some of the scientific concepts have therefore been simplified. However, I believe that the manual will also appeal to the practical men and women who make the everyday decisions on local strategy and tactics. Techniques of examination best applicable to field practice, methods of conducting population surveys, examining and dealing with the data generated, and approaches to control of both hookworm and hookworm anaemia are outlined.

A. Davis, M.D.
Formerly Director
Parasitic Diseases Programme
World Health Organization

Acknowledgements

The authors gratefully acknowledge the significant contributions made to this publication by Dr A. Davis, formerly Director, Parasitic Diseases Programme, World Health Organization, Geneva, Switzerland, Mr H. Dixon, Epidemiological and Statistical Methodology, World Health Organization, Geneva, Switzerland, Professor H. M. Gilles, Department of Pharmacology and Therapeutics, University of Liverpool, Liverpool, England, Dr J. M. Gurney, formerly of Nutrition, World Health Organization, Geneva, Switzerland, and Professor A. Rougemont, Faculty of Medicine, University of Geneva, Geneva, Switzerland. They also wish to thank Miss E. Certain, Miss M. A. Eddison and Miss P. A. Scarrott for their assistance.

Introduction

> **Hookworm infection and the iron deficiency
> it causes are still important health problems
> in many areas of the developing world**

About one quarter of the world's population has hookworm infection, one of the commonest of the soil-transmitted helminthiases. It is prevalent throughout the tropics and subtropics, wherever there is faecal contamination of the environment. Various figures have been published on the extent of infection; according to one source, for example, over 900 million people are infected worldwide (*1*), while another quotes 685 million people in south-east Asia, 132 million in Africa and 104 million in Central and South America (*2*). Although these estimates were made on the basis of meagre data, their importance lies in drawing attention to the magnitude of the problem of hookworm infection in relation to other diseases (*3*).

Two species of hookworm, *Ancylostoma duodenale* and *Necator americanus*, whose geographical distributions overlap, commonly infect humans. Prevalence rates vary widely with altitude, climate and ecological or human factors and may exceed 80% in certain areas.

Adult hookworms live in the duodenum and jejunum, attached to the intestinal mucosa from which they suck blood. The chronic blood loss this causes gradually depletes body iron stores, leading eventually to iron deficiency anaemia which may be widespread and often severe in an infected community. Hookworm infection can therefore be of major public health importance.

Complete eradication of hookworm infection in a community is feasible only with adequate sanitary disposal of faeces. It is, however, perfectly possible and obviously desirable to reduce hookworm loads in the population, thus keeping the prevalence and severity of hookworm-induced iron deficiency anaemia under control and significantly reducing morbidity and mortality.

Suitable approaches for evaluating the problem and achieving such control, based on present knowledge of the subject and the technology currently available, are described in this manual. It is hoped that the manual will be of use to those responsible for planning, organizing and supervising prevention and control activities.

> **Significant reductions in morbidity and**
> **mortality caused by hookworm infection**
> **are possible in many parts of the world**

1. Hookworms infecting humans

Two species of hookworm, *Ancylostoma duodenale* and *Necator americanus*, commonly parasitize and mature in humans. Other species, including the hookworms of cats and dogs, may also invade and develop to varying degrees in humans. For instance, *A. ceylanicum*, a parasite of cats and dogs, occasionally parasitizes humans, but those infected usually harbour only a few worms; *A. braziliense* may penetrate the skin but usually fails to migrate to deeper tissues and mature, and the same is probably true of *A. caninum* and *Uncinaria stenocephala*.

Identification of *A. duodenale* and *N. americanus*

The adult worms can be distinguished with a hand lens, without the need for a microscope. Males measure 5–11 mm and females 9–13 mm in length, with dorsally curved anterior ends. *N. americanus* is much more slender than *A. duodenale*, is more finely tapered in the anterior part, and has a distinct bend in the anterior tip (hence 'hook' worm). In contrast, the anterior part of *A. duodenale* tapers only slightly and its dorsal curve is relatively less marked. (See Fig. 1.)

Microscopic examination of the mouth opening on the ventral surface of a hookworm permits precise identification of the species. *A. duodenale* has two pairs of "teeth" whereas *N. americanus* has two curved cutting plates (see Fig. 2). The males may also be distinguished by differences in the structure of the copulatory bursa (see Annex 1).

The two species cannot be distinguished by microscopic examination of their eggs, which are very similar. However, hatching the eggs in faecal cultures allows the species of the emergent filariform larvae to be identified. (The identification of *A. duodenale* and *N. americanus* eggs, larvae and adults is described in more detail in Annex 1.)

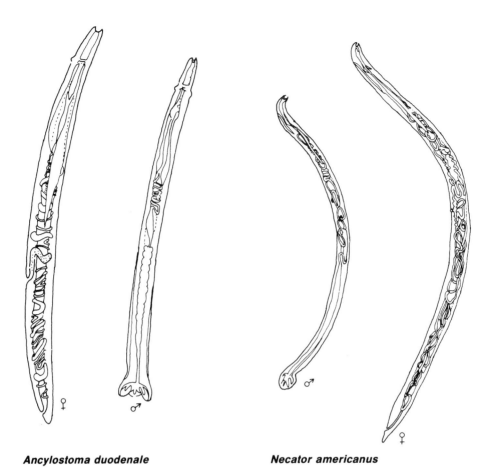

Ancylostoma duodenale   **Necator americanus**

Fig. 1. Adult hookworms of man

Redrawn from: BEAVER, P. C. & JUNG, R. C., ed. *Animal agents and vectors of human disease*, 5th ed. Philadelphia, Lea & Febiger, 1985.

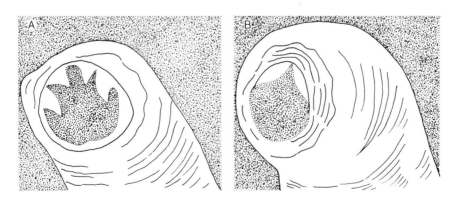

Fig. 2. Mouth openings of *Ancylostoma duodenale* (A) and *Necator americanus* (B)

(Note the teeth (A) or plates (B) for cutting tissue.)
Redrawn from: MARKELL, E. K. ET AL. *Medical parasitology.* Philadelphia, Saunders, 1986.

Geographical distribution

The geographical distribution of *A. duodenale* and *N. americanus* is shown in Fig. 3, in which the northern and southern limits are indicated.

In general, both species occur together, although *N. americanus* is the prevailing species throughout the tropics and subtropics. *A. duodenale* tends to prevail in cooler and drier climates, e.g. northern Africa and the eastern Mediterranean, parts of northern China, north-west India and southern Europe. Hookworms are rarely found, or occur only as light infections, in arid zones where the dry seasons are prolonged, or in temperate climates.

Life cycle of the hookworm

Mature female hookworms of the *A. duodenale* and *N. americanus* species produce between 5000 and 25000 eggs each day. Cell division begins during the passage of the eggs along the intestine, and by the time the eggs are passed in the faeces they are usually at the 4- or 8-celled stage. The eggs are not infective.

In warm, moist conditions outside the body, further development occurs with the formation of a first-stage (L_1) rhabditiform larva. At 25–35 °C, embryonation and hatching of L_1 larvae occur in 24 hours. Development is slower at lower temperatures, and at 15 °C hatching does not occur until the fifth day. At higher temperatures (up to 40 °C)

Table 1. Effect of temperature on hookworm eggs and larvae

Temperature	Species	Effect on eggs and larvae
Above 45 °C	A. duodenale	Larvae killed in 90 minutes
	N. americanus	Larvae killed in 15 minutes
45 °C	A. duodenale	Most eggs fail to hatch
40 °C	N. americanus	
15–35 °C	A. duodenale	90% of eggs hatch in 24 hours
20–35 °C	N. americanus	
20–27 °C	A. duodenale	Ideal temperatures for larvae
28–32 °C	N. americanus	
15 °C	A. duodenale	90% of eggs hatch in 5 days
	N. americanus	Fewer eggs hatch

5

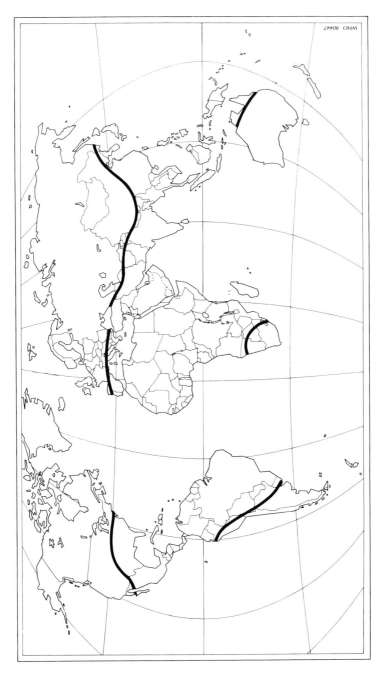

Fig. 3. Distribution of *Ancylostoma duodenale* and *Necator americanus*

WHO 90447

development also slows down. Some 90% of *A. duodenale* and *N. americanus* eggs will hatch in the temperature ranges 15–35 °C and 20–35 °C, respectively. The former fail to hatch above 45 °C and the latter above 40 °C. (See Table 1.)

The free-living rhabditiform larvae that emerge from the eggs are about 0.2 mm long, live in faeces or in soil polluted with faeces, and feed on faecal bacteria and other organic matter. They develop into second stage (L_2) larvae, which continue to feed actively and grow but are not yet infective. The largest of these larvae measure up to 0.5 mm in length and are just visible when suspended in clear water and viewed in good light against a dark background.

About five days after hatching, feeding ceases and the non-infective rhabditiform (L_2) larvae develop into non-feeding invasive filariform (L_3) larvae, 0.5–0.7 mm in length. These are very active and migrate upwards on to low vegetation as far as the moisture film extends or downwards into the most superficial layers of the soil.

The invasive larvae will penetrate human skin on contact. All *N. americanus* infections occur in this way; infection with *A. duodenale* may also be acquired by ingestion of filariform larvae present in water or on moist raw vegetables.

Hookworm infection is acquired mainly by skin contact with contaminated soil or vegetation

---

After penetrating the skin, usually between the toes or on the legs and buttocks, the filariform larvae enter the circulation and are carried to the lungs. There they leave the blood vessels, pass through the walls of the alveoli and migrate up the bronchioles, bronchi, and trachea to reach the pharynx. On being swallowed, they enter the stomach and the upper part of the small intestine.

Once in the duodenum and jejunum, the larvae develop further, becoming fourth-stage (L_4) larvae equipped with a temporary buccal capsule and capable of feeding on the intestinal mucosa and blood. This temporary capsule is shed with the cuticle when the larvae moult to become adult hookworms.

The migration of hookworm larvae through the body to the intestine takes 3–5 days. About 6–8 weeks after penetrating the skin, the hookworms reach maturity and eggs start appearing in the faeces (see Fig. 4.)

Infective *A. duodenale* larvae ingested in food or water do not migrate through the lungs but settle directly in the small intestine. However, some larvae become arrested in their development and remain in a dormant state in the tissues (muscles or intestines) for an extended time (up to 200

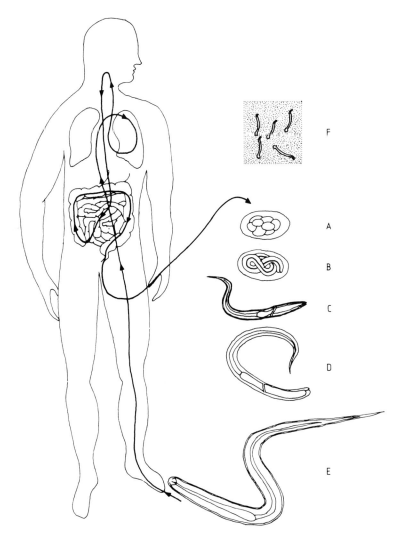

Fig. 4. Life cycle of *Ancylostoma duodenale* and *Necator americanus*

A = hookworm egg in faeces
B = embryonating egg
C + D = rhabditiform larvae (L_1, L_2)
E = filariform, infective larva (L_3)
F = L_4 larvae and adult hookworms attached to jejunal mucosa

days) before resuming growth and becoming mature. In such cases, the prepatent period—between infection and the appearance of eggs in the faeces—may last several months.

It has been suggested, though not confirmed, that *A. duodenale* in the tissues may be a source of transmammary infection, causing neonatal ancylostomiasis.

2. Clinical pathology of hookworm infection

In the early stages of hookworm infection, symptoms, signs and pathological changes are transient and attributable to the penetration of the skin by larvae, to the subsequent migration of larvae through the lungs and to intestinal mucosal injury. In established infections, symptoms and signs are due mainly to anaemia and hypoproteinaemia.

Penetration of the skin

When the invasive filariform larvae penetrate the skin they may cause a stinging sensation, followed by irritation, erythema, oedema and a papulovesicular eruption – the so-called ground itch. These symptoms rarely occur in people who live in areas endemic for the hookworms specific to man, but may be noted in visitors from non-endemic areas. Itching and dermatitis are usually more marked in zoonotic hookworm infections (e.g. with *A. caninum* or *A. braziliense*).

Migration of larvae

The migration of hookworm larvae through the body causes few pathological changes, but small haemorrhages and leukocytic or eosinophilic infiltrations may occur where larvae pass through the alveolar walls of the lungs. Migration of larvae through the respiratory tract may cause coughing, due to irritation of the bronchial and tracheal mucous membranes.

Established intestinal infection

In the duodenum and jejunum, hookworms attach themselves to the intestine by engulfing a part of the intestinal mucosa in their buccal cavities (see Fig. 5). There they feed on blood from cut vessels and on

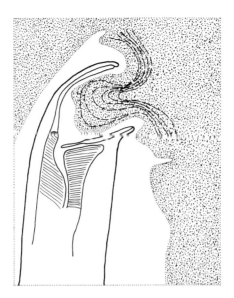

Fig. 5. Hookworm attached to mucosa of small intestine

Redrawn from photomicrograph by the Armed Forces Institute of Pathology, Washington, DC.

mucosal tissue. At the points of attachment there is usually some bleeding and inflammatory reaction, but these minute lesions heal quickly when hookworms move to other sites, which they do every 4–6 hours.

During the intestinal phase, those infected may have epigastric duodenal-type pain, indigestion, loss of appetite or diarrhoea. There may be marked eosinophilia, but this is unusual. However, such symptoms and signs are common to many complaints and it may therefore be difficult to attribute them with certainty to hookworm infection. In areas where hookworm is prevalent, a high incidence of "duodenal ulcer", reported by hospitals and health centres but not clinically confirmed, may in fact be a reflection of hookworm infection.

Chronic blood loss

The most serious consequence of hookworm infection is chronic blood loss from the duodenum and jejunum. If the infection is not adequately treated blood loss may continue for many years, leading to depletion of body iron stores and the development of iron deficiency anaemia. There is also loss of serum proteins, which may result in severe hypo-albuminaemia.

Whether or not a person with hookworm infection develops anaemia depends on several factors, including the species of hookworm, the worm load, the duration of infection, body iron stores, dietary iron intake and absorption, and physiological iron requirements.

Hookworm infections may be classified into two main groups:

- infection with *little or no anaemia*
- infection with *iron deficiency anaemia*

The distinction is of great public health importance in deciding which control measures are most suitable for an infected population.

Symptoms and signs of hookworm anaemia

In chronic infections, symptoms and signs are mainly those associated with anaemia and hypoalbuminaemia. If the anaemia is gradual in onset, which is usually the case, symptoms may be relatively slight, even when haemoglobin levels are very low. Patients may complain of general weakness, of being easily fatigued, of difficulty in doing a full day's work and of shortness of breath on exertion. Palpitation, dizziness, epigastric pain (which may disappear after anthelminthic treatment), aching of the legs which is unrelated to exercise, and loss of appetite are common symptoms; men may also complain of impotence. In a few patients, there may be precordial or anginal pain, blurred vision, ringing in the ears, difficulty in swallowing, tingling sensations in the hands, or swelling of the ankles.

In addition to pallor of the skin, conjunctivae, tongue and buccal mucosa, patients may have increased pulse pressure, peripheral vasodilation and increased venous pressure. Koilonychia (flattening and concavity of the fingernails) and angular stomatitis, which are common in iron deficiency anaemia, may be present and there may be retinal haemorrhages. Most patients report having had symptoms for only relatively short periods, usually 2–3 months and rarely as long as a year.

Despite the degree of anaemia, most patients do not appear to be really ill. A minority, however, both look and feel ill, have a slow pulse, collapsed veins, low body temperature (below 36 °C), severe oedema (often affecting the face and arms as well as the legs) and ascites. The oedema has been attributed to hypoalbuminaemia rather than to the heart failure which may be present. A type of skin pallor that accompanies hypoalbuminaemia has also been described and responds only slowly to anthelminthic treatment.

Children with hookworm anaemia may suffer from impaired physical development, apathy, irritability, listlessness and poor academic performance in school. Pica, a craving to eat non-food substances, including soil, may also be observed.

3. Hookworm infection as a cause of anaemia

That hookworm can cause severe and widespread anaemia was first demonstrated, beyond all doubt and on a very large scale, in 1880, during the construction of the St Gotthard Tunnel through the Alps. Many thousands of workers were affected and morbidity and mortality were high. Proof that infection with *Ancylostoma duodenale* was responsible also provided the explanation of miner's anaemia, which was prevalent in many European countries at the time.

Given high ambient temperature and humidity plus unhygienic conditions, such as existed in mines in temperate zones and still exist in plantations in the tropics and subtropics, hookworm disease may assume *epidemic* proportions in a labour force if it is not kept under control. In such environments, however, recognition, treatment and prevention of the disease should present little difficulty.

The situation is very different in areas where hookworm infection is *endemic* but where transmission and intensity of infection are more moderate in degree. In these circumstances, which are found in much of the developing world, cause and effect relationships are less clearcut, and the relative importance of the various contributory factors may be difficult to assess.

> **The most serious consequence of hookworm infection
> is chronic blood loss from the small intestine
> leading to the development of iron deficiency anaemia**

Iron balance

Large numbers of the world's population live in a state of precarious iron balance, because of either low dietary iron intake or low intestinal absorption of dietary iron. For such people, any chronic blood loss, however slight, may be sufficient to exhaust body iron stores and induce iron deficiency anaemia. This is often the case where rice is the staple food, little meat is eaten, dietary ascorbic acid is low and a high intake of tannates (in tea for example) impairs iron absorption. Relatively small hookworm loads, which would usually be considered harmless, may precipitate severe anaemia in children and in women of childbearing age, whose physiological needs for iron are high.

In other parts of the world, where more animal protein is consumed and dietary iron is relatively high and well absorbed, hookworm anaemia is associated only with much greater intensity of infection.

It is therefore unwise to generalize by stating that hookworm anaemia occurs only with worm loads above a certain level: due consideration must be given to the various factors that determine iron balance in a given population.

Development of hookworm anaemia depends on:

- **the host** — **iron balance, body iron stores, dietary iron, absorption of iron, physiological requirements, other iron losses**
- **the parasite** — **hookworm species, hookworm load, duration of infection.**

Body iron stores

Body iron comprises two main parts—metabolically active iron (in haemoglobin, myoglobin and various enzymes) which is required for normal function and storage iron (in ferritin and haemosiderin) which constitutes a reserve upon which the body can draw. Women during their reproductive years have lower iron stores than men. As they generally

Table 2. Examples of body iron status in adults in a developing country

Type of iron	Body iron concentration (mg/kg)		Total body iron (mg)	
	men	women	man (60 kg)	woman (50 kg)
Metabolically active iron	37	33	2 220	1 650
Storage iron	13	5	780	250
Total body iron	50	38	3 000	1 900

weigh less, their iron reserves may be less than one-third of those in men and may even be completely depleted. Examples are given in Table 2.

Iron absorption

Absorption of iron for maintenance of body iron stores depends on the amount of iron in the diet, the type of iron and its availability, the presence of factors that enhance or inhibit iron absorption, the health of the individual and the status of body iron stores. As iron reserves diminish, absorption increases. The availability of iron from grains and vegetables is enhanced by the presence of ascorbic acid or meat (including fish and poultry), while increased intestinal motility, such as may occur with a bulky diet or during an episode of diarrhoea, may interfere with absorption. Part of the iron in the blood lost into the intestine in hookworm infection is reabsorbed.

Dietary iron

Dietary iron is derived from animal (haem iron) and vegetable (non-haem iron) sources. Haem iron is readily available to the body; non-haem iron is much less readily available and its absorption is highly dependent on the overall composition of a meal. Despite the fact that meat is an important component of the diet in industrialized countries, iron deficiency is not uncommon and it has been found necessary to fortify wheat flour with iron. Even so, some 20% of women of reproductive age are deficient in iron.

In developing countries, the situation is much more serious. Meat, fish, poultry and eggs are eaten in only small amounts, if at all, by the poorer sections of the population. A diet that is almost entirely of vegetable origin may provide as little as 5–10 mg of iron per day—mostly non-haem iron—of which only a small fraction may be available for absorption because of losses during cooking, the presence of substances that inhibit absorption (phosphates, phytates, tannates), and a low intake of ascorbic acid. Such a diet is barely sufficient to meet normal physiological iron needs (estimated at 0.5–1.0 mg per day for men and children and 1.0–2.0 mg per day for women of reproductive age and adolescents) and is clearly inadequate to supply the 2.0–4.8 mg per day required in pregnancy.

Blood and iron losses in hookworm infection

Blood loss in hookworm infection has been estimated as 0.20 ml per worm per day (range 0.14–0.26 ml) for *A. duodenale* and 0.04 ml per worm per

Table 3. Estimated blood and iron losses in hookworm infection

	A. duodenale		N. americanus	
	Mean	Range	Mean	Range
Daily blood loss, ml/worm	0.20	0.14–0.26	0.04	0.02–0.07
No. of worms causing blood loss of 1 ml/day	5	4–7	25	14–50
Daily egg production, per female worm		10 000–25 000		5 000–10 000
At 1 000 eggs/g of faeces[a]:				
Estimated hookworm load[b]	11 (5 F, 6 M)		32 (13 F, 19 M)	
Blood loss, ml/day	2.2	1.54–2.86	1.3	0.82–2.24
Iron loss, mg/day[c]	0.76		0.45	

[a] Based on stool weight of 135 g.
[b] At 25 000 eggs/day for A. duodenale and 10 000 eggs/day for N. americanus.
[c] Based on a haemoglobin level of 100 g/litre of blood.

day (range 0.02–0.07 ml) for *N. americanus* (see Table 3). However, the arithmetic relationships between hookworm load, egg counts and blood losses are difficult to estimate reliably since they are affected by the following variables:

- Intensity of infection. A female *A. duodenale* produces 10 000–25 000 eggs per day and a female *N. americanus* 5 000–10 000 eggs per day; egg production is higher in light infections.
- The concentration of eggs per gram of faeces, which varies with the weight and consistency of faeces produced (from 70 g/day in a child to 135 g/day or more in an adult).
- The ratio of *A. duodenale* to *N. americanus* in mixed infections.
- The sex ratio of the hookworms, which is about 1.5 males to 1 female in *N. americanus* infections and 1 : 1 in *A. duodenale* infections.

With these reservations, it may be roughly calculated that 1000 eggs per gram of faeces represents a worm load of about 11 *A. duodenale* or 32 *N. americanus* and a daily blood loss of 2.2 and 1.3 ml respectively.

Over a period, even small hookworm loads may cause sufficient blood loss to deplete body iron reserves. For example, a blood loss of 1 ml per day (equivalent to 0.347 mg of iron at a haemoglobin level of 100 g/litre of blood) would cause a loss of 250 mg of iron in 2 years, or the equivalent of the total body iron stores in a woman of 50 kg (see Table 4).

Table 4. Depletion of body iron stores by low hookworm loads

| | Daily blood loss | |
	1 ml	5 ml
Causative no. of hookworms:		
A. duodenale	5	25
N. americanus	22	110
Blood Hb 120 g/litre:		
Daily iron loss	0.416 mg	2.082 mg
Time to lose 250 mg iron[a]	600 days	120 days
Blood Hb 100 g/litre:		
Daily iron loss	0.347 mg	1.735 mg
Time to lose 250 mg iron[a]	720 days	144 days

[a] Estimated body iron store in a woman weighing 50 kg.

In people whose dietary intake of iron is low and whose body iron stores are already depleted, heavy hookworm loads can give rise to iron deficiency anaemia within just a few weeks.

Where dietary iron intake is low, just a few hookworms active over a short period of time may be sufficient to cause iron deficiency anaemia, especially in women and children.

Even normal levels of dietary iron will not protect against anaemia in the presence of a high hookworm load.

---

4. Epidemiology of hookworm infection

Climatic factors affecting transmission

In areas where both temperature and rainfall are generally suitable for the development of hookworm larvae, the intensity of infection may show marked regional or local differences because of climatic factors. Even where the total annual rainfall appears adequate for intensive hookworm transmission, infections may be light if the rainfall is seasonal, lasting only a few months. For any month to be favourable for transmission, about 100 mm of evenly distributed rainfall is required, i.e. 9–10 rainy days per month, other ecological conditions being suitable.

Heavy infections may occur in arid zones, on arable land or fruit and vegetable farms, if irrigation provides enough soil moisture (for instance, in north Africa, the eastern Mediterranean, northwestern India). If hookworm development takes place underground, infections may also occur in regions which would otherwise be too dry or too cold; examples include mines and tunnels, where humidity and temperature may be relatively high.

**Climate sets the general limits of
distribution of hookworm infection,
but local prevalence and intensity are
largely determined by human activities**

Distribution of infective larvae

Under natural tropical conditions, the free-living larvae are short-lived. The first two feeding stages, the rhabditiform (L_1, L_2) larvae, remain in the faeces or faecally polluted soil and are not very mobile. Many die in the first few days while developing to the infective stage, most being ingested by predacious nematodes, mites and other invertebrates in the soil.

By contrast, the non-feeding, third stage (L_3), infective larvae are capable of considerable vertical movement (1 m or more), although they do not move far laterally. They migrate to the soil surface or to low vegetation in order to make contact with humans, and are therefore vulnerable to desiccation. They will exhaust their small food reserves and die quickly if forced to migrate up and down vegetation to avoid drying out; most live only a few days and few survive more than a month. The dispersion of hookworm eggs and larvae is summarized in Fig. 6.

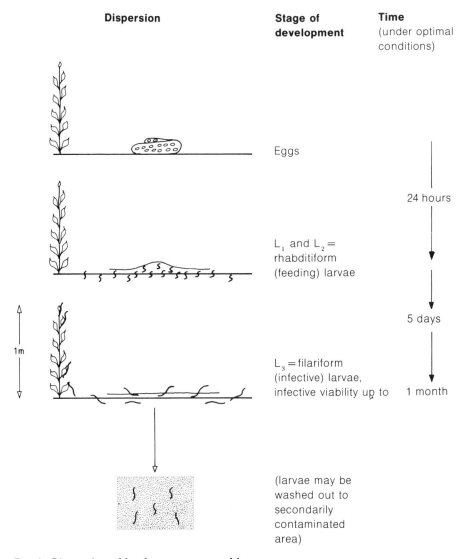

Fig. 6. Dispersion of hookworm eggs and larvae

Larval development and survival are favoured by shade, moisture, loamy soil, and vegetation; even grass will provide sufficient shade for a hookworm larva. Unshaded open areas, saline soils, rapidly draining sandy soils and compacted and waterlogged soils are all unfavourable for hookworm larvae. In general, primarily contaminated areas are limited to defecation grounds and fields fertilized with human faeces.

Larvae are not easily displaced by rainfall but very heavy rain may wash them from the original place of faecal deposition to another site. Torrential scouring rains may flush large numbers of hookworm larvae from latrines or faecally contaminated areas into ponds, pools or larger bodies of water. Heavy infection probably occurs in these secondarily contaminated areas.

Patterns of transmission

In an appropriate climate, the following conditions will together ensure the maintenance and spread of hookworm infection in a community:

● lack of sanitation and indiscriminate defecation by villagers, inhabitants of a peri-urban area, or a labour force; and

● use of inadequately composted human excreta as fertilizer.

The following are the three main epidemiological patterns of transmission (summarized in Table 5):

● Endemic hookworm infection in rural villages or peri-urban areas is caused essentially by the lack of sanitation and the use of nearby

Table 5. Major patterns of transmission of hookworm infection

Pattern of transmission	Site of most active transmission	Highest prevalence and intensity
Endemic Due to lack of sanitation (rural or peri-urban)	Defecation areas on wasteland near houses	Older children, women, elderly people
Endemic Related to small-scale agriculture (rural)	Fields and vegetable plots manured with human faeces	Men, women, children working in fields
Epidemic – focal Related to agriculture or specific occupations	Plantations and farms, mines and tunnels	Labourers and farmers, miners and tunnel workers

wasteland for defecation. All sections of the community may be affected, with the highest prevalence and intensity of infection concentrated in those who spend much of their time in the village and who visit the contaminated area most frequently (generally older children, adolescents, women and elderly people).

- Endemic hookworm infection in rural villages may also be related to the use of human faeces as manure on agricultural plots; those most affected are the family members who tend these plots.

- Epidemic or focal outbreaks of hookworm infection may occur on plantations and among farm labourers, miners and tunnel workers exposed to high levels of infection under conditions that are particularly favourable for transmission.

In practice, the first and second patterns of transmission commonly coexist in rural communities. In agricultural exposure to infection, rural sociological factors, such as the type of work done, determine the groups at greatest risk. For example, if adult women do the harvesting, as in tea plantations, they will harbour the heavy infections; if men plough the nightsoil into the fields, they will be the group at special risk.

How much hookworm infection is associated with inadequate rural or peri-urban sanitation and how much with agricultural activity has to be established locally, by studying the distribution of infection among the population, local defecation behaviour and agricultural practices.

Defecation behaviour

Because hookworm larvae do not disperse laterally, heavy infection is usually acquired in the immediate vicinity of faecal deposition—in defecation grounds outside villages, at the edges of fields or in plantations.

The desire for privacy during defecation makes people tend to choose areas under or concealed by bushes, which are likely to be moist and shaded and therefore provide favourable conditions for the development of hookworm larvae. The habitual use of the same area for defecation leads to heavy faecal pollution and the constant risk of reinfection. Hookworm larvae may also occur near footpaths, by the roadside or, in peri-urban areas, in playgrounds, all of which may be sources of infection.

Agricultural activities

Heavy hookworm infection is associated with the growing of certain crops, including coffee beans, jasmine flowers, mulberry leaves, sugarcane and tea. Generally speaking, crops that provide shade (or are cultivated in the shade of taller trees) and are grown on loamy soils (a mixture of sand, clay and silt that holds moisture but does not become waterlogged) provide good conditions for transmission of hookworm infection.

Irrigation permits hookworm infection to occur in areas that would otherwise be too dry for larvae to survive. However, hookworm eggs and larvae develop poorly in standing water or compacted, waterlogged soil; crops grown in flooded fields (e.g. rice, jute) are therefore rarely associated with intense infection, even if the flooding is intermittent.

Labour-intensive agricultural activities, whether concerned with planting, cultivating or harvesting, tend to perpetuate hookworm infection. When a large labour force is in the field for long periods daily, far from sanitary facilities, heavy faecal pollution of the soil is inevitable. Penetration of the skin by infective larvae is facilitated where labourers customarily work barefoot.

Use of human excreta as manure

The use of fresh or inadequately composted human faeces as manure may contribute significantly to hookworm transmission. Digging faeces into the soil breaks up both the soil and the faecal mass and thus encourages embryonation, hatching and larval development. Moreover, treading the faeces into the soil ensures prolonged skin contact with infective larvae from previous faecal deposition.

However, thoroughly composted faeces or faeces mixed with urine and kept for some time do not present this risk. The addition of certain chemical fertilizers will also kill hookworm eggs and larvae and, at the same time, improve the quality of the manure.

Distribution of infection in a community

In areas where the overall prevalence of hookworm infection in the population is low, there may be certain localities or population groups in which many people are infected. Conversely, where prevalence is generally high, certain villages or sections of the community may have relatively low rates of infection.

The intensity of infection also varies widely between individuals and between groups in a given community. While many people may be infected, most will have only light infections and only a few will be heavily infected. For example, 60% or more of the total hookworm load in an area may be carried by less than 10% of the infected population.

An example of the variation in intensity and distribution of hookworm infection in a community is given in Fig. 7. The reasons (behavioural,

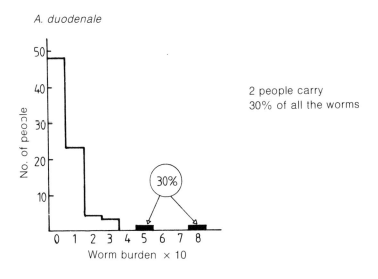

A. duodenale

2 people carry
30% of all the worms

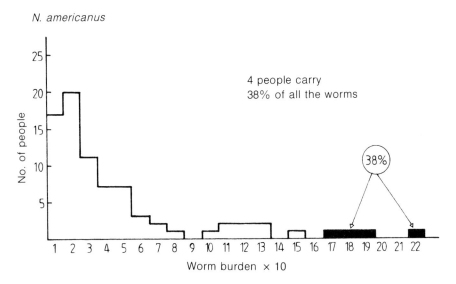

N. americanus

4 people carry
38% of all the worms

Fig. 7. The intensity distribution of hookworm infections in an Iranian village

After CROLL, N. A. & GHADIRIAN, E. Wormy persons: contributions to the nature and patterns of overdispersion with *Ascaris lumbricoides, Ancylostoma duodenale, Necator americanus* and *Trichuris trichiura. Tropical and geographical medicine,* **33**: 241–248 (1981).

genetic, social) for these individual differences are not fully understood. However, variations in prevalence and intensity of infection with sex, race and age reflect the degree of exposure to infection of the groups concerned and are mainly related to agricultural occupations and defecation habits.

Hookworm infection is usually endemic, with prevalence gradually increasing during childhood, reaching a maximum value in adolescence and early adult life and remaining stable or decreasing slowly thereafter. Sometimes, prevalence rises again in older people who use defecation grounds near their homes.

On average, adult *A. duodenale* and *N. americanus* live for about one year and four years respectively. The maintenance of hookworm infection prevalence rates and intensity levels in a community, therefore, represents a balance between the constant loss of hookworms and reinfection. Where contamination of the soil and exposure to reinfection can be reduced, the level of infection will tend to decrease with time.

> **Most of the total hookworm load in an infected community is usually carried by a relatively small section of the population**

Morbidity and mortality

In rural areas of the tropics and subtropics, where there is little or no sanitation, the prevalence of hookworm infection in a country may vary considerably, from 10–20% in the drier zones to 80–90% where humidity and rainfall are high. Both patterns may be associated with severe degrees of iron deficiency anaemia.

High prevalence of hookworm infection does not necessarily mean that anaemia will be an important public health problem in a community. Similarly, where hookworm prevalence is low, severe anaemia may still be found in many individuals or in certain sections of the population. The crucial factor is the balance between iron absorbed from food, physiological iron requirements and iron loss due to hookworm infection.

Table 6. Hookworm infection and associated morbidity and mortality

	Japan, 1950s Agricultural workers	El Salvador, 1970s General population
Population	35 000 000	5 700 000
Infected with hookworm	10 000 000	2 000 000
	(approx. 30%)	(35%)
Incapacitated by anaemia	1 000 000	4 000[a]
Deaths each year	1 000	1 000

[a] With blood haemoglobin levels below 50 g/litre.

Each situation has to be evaluated locally. In areas where hookworm anaemia is present, 50% or more of the population may have haemoglobin values below the normal range and some of these may have severe degrees of anaemia.

In general, morbidity and mortality rates due to hookworm infection are low but, because so many millions are affected, total deaths (estimated at 50 000 to 60 000 a year) and numbers of patients attending health services (1.5 million a year) are relatively high. Two large-scale surveys, one from the early 1950s concerning agricultural workers in Japan (4) and the other, published in 1978, relating to the general population of El Salvador, (5), gave estimates of morbidity and mortality associated with hookworm infection. (See Table 6.) In Japan, the problem was essentially one of morbidity in an adult labour force, whereas in El Salvador, the high mortality rate among infected children was relatively much more important.

5. Principles of prevention and control

With economic progress, hookworm anaemia has disappeared from many areas, but is still a formidable problem in much of the world. Measures to control hookworm anaemia produce striking results, and the lessons learned from programmes started more than 50 years ago are still valid. A well managed programme may encourage community cooperation in hookworm control and also promote intersectoral collaboration in other areas. Implementing control measures within other programmes will keep costs and the need for supporting infrastructure to a minimum.

Control of hookworm anaemia is a gradual process; an effective and comprehensive programme requires a series of well thought-out measures, implemented in small steps. In many circumstances, it may be a vital component of a general strategy for the control of anaemia, involving supplemental iron, dietary education and fortification of foods with iron, as well as specific antiparasite measures.

Lessons from past control programmes

The first attempt to control hookworm disease on a global scale was initiated by the Rockefeller Foundation in 1913 and continued into the 1920s and 1930s, reaching 52 countries. This campaign established the following basic principles for hookworm control.

- A distinction must be made between hookworm infection and hookworm disease. (The term "hookworm disease" always denotes the presence of moderate, marked or severe iron deficiency anaemia associated with, and due to, hookworm infection.)
- Massive infection from a single or occasional exposure to hookworm-infected soil is rare.
- Sanitation alone will control hookworm infection and disease but this method is extremely slow.
- Hookworm disease can quickly be brought under control by mass treatment of heavily infected people.

Much of what was learned from the broad experience in this campaign is still valid. In Japan, the prevalence of hookworm infection fell as a result of a national parasite control programme from 23.2% in 1922 to 0.01% in 1984. Hookworm infection has also been eradicated from coal mines and tunnel works in Europe, and greatly reduced in fruit and vegetable plantations in Italy.

Hookworm disease was a major public health problem in the south-eastern United States in the first two decades of this century, with prevalence rates in rural areas ranging from 20% to 60%. The current regional prevalence is unknown but in Georgia, one of the most severely affected states, the prevalence of infection in the northern part of the state has decreased from about 20% in 1911–1914, to about 7% in 1961–1964 and 0.3% in 1970. Corresponding figures for the central area of the state are 50%, 10% and 4%, and for the warm, humid southern part 60%, 13% and 6%. Prevalence has since declined even further, but small foci of low prevalence remain in some economically depressed areas where climate, soil type and primitive sanitary facilities provide ideal conditions for the parasite's survival.

Although there are no exact data on the global incidence of hookworm anaemia, a marked decrease has been observed in some developing countries where sanitation and health services have been improved, while in many others, both prevalence and intensity of hookworm infection— and even mortality rates—have remained almost unchanged.

Effect of improved living standards

A general rise in the standard of living has played a major role in the spontaneous decline of severe hookworm infection in areas where it was once prevalent but is now rare. Many factors have contributed to this, their relative importance depending on whether transmission occurred mainly in the immediate vicinity of houses or further away in fields and plantations.

In peri-urban and urban areas, the introduction of sanitary latrines, piped water supply and effective drainage will reduce the prevalence and intensity of hookworm infection, as will a water-borne sewerage system and a properly carried out rehousing programme. Housing design may be very important, particularly if it encourages the use of sanitation facilities and discourages indiscriminate defecation. In this connection, the planning and maintenance of outdoor spaces and play areas and even the location of windows overlooking them may have significant beneficial effects. Food-borne infection is also likely to be reduced by the provision of water for washing vegetables.

Where living standards are improved, shoes are more widely worn, even in agricultural areas, and provide significant protection against infective larvae. Greater prosperity is also generally associated with a decline in the use of natural manures, an increase in the use of chemical fertilizers and the introduction of mechanization in agriculture. As a result, faecal contamination of the soil is reduced, fewer working hours are spent in the fields, and exposure of the individual to direct contact with soil or crops that harbour infective larvae is thus lessened.

Hookworm anaemia remains a major problem

Despite improvements in much of the world, hookworm infection and the iron deficiency anaemia it causes are still major public health problems in several areas of the tropics and subtropics, and continue to affect many millions of people. Often, the severity and extent of the problems are not fully appreciated. Because they are most prevalent in rural areas, where health facilities are generally very limited and of poor quality, hookworm infection and anaemia may be under-diagnosed and under-reported; as a consequence, inadequate measures for treatment, control and prevention may be a major factor in their persistence in the community.

In these circumstances, hookworm anaemia may also remain unrecognized as an underlying cause of high maternal morbidity and mortality, apathy and poor health in children, and easy fatiguability and impaired working capacity in adults. Its effects are insidious. Once the relationship is suspected, however, confirmation presents little difficulty and the discovery of iron deficiency anaemia in one area should lead to a search for it in other areas and adequate measures for its control in all sections of the affected community.

In areas where malaria is endemic, it is important to take this into account as a cause of anaemia in the population, both in assessing the relationship between haemoglobin levels and hookworm loads and in planning measures to control anaemia.

Objectives and options in control of hookworm anaemia

The first priority in control of hookworm anaemia is to reduce mortality and morbidity as rapidly as possible. Success in this requires all anaemic people in the community to be treated with iron and anthelminthics. In programme terms, this means adopting or adapting one of the measures outlined in Table 7—standard case management, targeted treatment, mass treatment and supplementary iron distribution.

The longer-term objective, reduction in the overall intensity and prevalence of hookworm infection, requires improvements in hygiene and

Table 7. Specific measures to control hookworm anaemia

Epidemiological pattern	Appropriate measure
Anaemia common but no special pattern	*Standard case management* Iron and anthelminthic treatment of all those with anaemia
Certain groups particularly affected	*Targeted treatment* Iron and anthelminthic treatment of all anaemic or infected people in the group
Majority of the community affected, with many severely anaemic	*Mass treatment* Anthelminthic treatment of all members of the community to reduce worm loads; iron treatment of those with moderate to severe anaemia
Mild to moderate anaemia common, but hookworm loads generally low	*Supplementary iron* Distribution of small doses of iron to those at special risk; fortification of a basic food with iron

Table 8. Basic approach to control of hookworm anaemia

	Programme objectives		
	Mortality reduction	**Morbidity reduction**	**Prevalence reduction**
Time frame	Weeks	Months	Years
Priority	High	Medium	Low
Target population	Individuals	Special groups	Communities
Health service responsibility	Primary health care Health centres Hospitals	Primary health care Health centres Maternal and child health Schools Occupational health	Public health service −special programmes −sanitation unit −health education
Measures available	Standard case management	Standard case management Targeted or mass treatment Sanitation Health education	Iron supplements Sanitation Health education

sanitation (particularly the disposal of faeces) and health education of all sections of the community. With the cooperation of the local population, this phase of the programme may be realized at affordable cost.

A combined programme, involving the regular treatment of those with hookworm anaemia (usually the most heavily infected), the introduction of sanitation, and health education, is the ideal approach to controlling hookworm anaemia and limiting the spread of hookworm infection. The main elements of such an approach are summarized in Table 8.

Standard case management

Standard case management with iron and anthelminthic therapy is the foundation of hookworm anaemia control. It can be applied on a large or small scale and is easy to organize and supervise. Rapid results are produced, the benefits of which are quickly appreciated by all in the community; the confidence this inspires is essential if sustained cooperation is to be obtained. The details of standard case management may be adapted to local conditions provided that the oral iron is given over a long enough period to allow body iron stores to be replenished and that a second anthelminthic is given at the end of iron treatment to prevent early relapse.

Standard case management may be used at all levels of health services—at the primary level, in health centres and hospitals, and in maternal and child health, school and occupational health services.

As the people with hookworm anaemia tend to be those with the highest hookworm loads in the community, their regular treatment with anthelminthics should contribute significantly to reducing the hookworm population in the area.

In summary, standard case management with iron and anthelminthic therapy:

- comprises three oral ferrous sulfate tablets daily for two months and one tablet daily for another four months, with an anthelminthic at the beginning and at the end of treatment
- is essential in all cases of hookworm anaemia
- quickly raises haemoglobin levels
- reduces mortality and morbidity
- reduces hookworm loads and blood loss
- replenishes body iron stores (if iron therapy is prolonged)
- is inexpensive, highly effective, and without risk
- can be used in villages and at any level of health services.

31

Targeted treatment

In some areas, relatively small groups of the population may be particularly exposed to hookworm infection. These groups may carry the largest hookworm loads and have the highest prevalence of severe hookworm anaemia within their communities. Where such high-risk groups can be identified, and where the rest of the population is relatively unaffected by hookworm anaemia, targeted treatment allows limited resources to be used to maximum effect.

Targeted treatment employs a standard type of management but is applied to groups of people rather than to individuals. As not all members of a 'target group' may be anaemic or harbour a heavy hookworm load at a given moment, targeted treatment may be restricted to those within the group who are actually anaemic; the screening test for anaemia is simple and inexpensive.

In other areas, provided that there is appropriate quantitative background information, treatment may be targeted according to a profile describing those likely to be heavily infected. In the southern United States, for example, it was recognized that most cases of hookworm disease (as distinct from infection) occurred in large, poor families in rural areas with sandy loam soils. Hookworm control programmes were therefore concentrated in those regions and were implemented on a household basis. 'Hookworm families' were identified by school-based stool surveys or by the recognition of anaemia in schoolchildren.

Where feasible, it may be advisable to administer anthelminthics as preventive treatment to people who are moving from endemic areas into areas where there is no hookworm infection, in order to ensure that the parasites do not become established. Examples include migrant agricultural workers, refugees and other displaced groups. People who are going to be rehoused, particularly children who may otherwise contaminate initially safe open areas such as yards and play areas, should also be considered for preventive anthelminthic treatment.

Mass treatment

Mass anthelminthic therapy aims to treat all members of a community during a relatively short period of time without examining them individually and irrespective of whether or not they are infected. It may be used when infection is so prevalent and intensive that almost everyone may be assumed to be infected and to contribute significantly to the continued existence of parasites in the community.

This approach has been successful where its cost is not prohibitive and where the population to be treated is cooperative (e.g. Japan, the

32

Republic of Korea). It is also successful when strong persuasion can be brought to bear on individuals who would otherwise avoid treatment. In the absence of sanitation, however, reinfection will occur and periodic retreatment will be necessary, which increases the expense. This approach is therefore not very practical in most poor countries.

Thus, large-scale anthelminthic treatment (without iron):

- reduces hookworm loads and blood loss
- prevents the development of anaemia in those not already anaemic
- does not replace the iron that has been lost
- does not produce a rise in haemoglobin levels
- in the absence of adequate sanitation, needs to be repeated every 6–12 months to keep hookworm loads low and is therefore costly
- may be cheaper as a targeted treatment than as a mass treatment.

Supplementary iron therapy

Even in patients with severe hookworm anaemia, treatment with oral iron alone brings about rapid improvement and raises haemoglobin to near-normal levels without anthelminthic therapy. Unless anthelminthic therapy is also given, however, haemoglobin levels in such patients will remain satisfactory only so long as iron supplements are maintained and will fall when iron is withdrawn.

Where hookworm infections are relatively light and dietary iron intake is low, the health problem is essentially one of widespread mild to moderate iron deficiency anaemia. In these circumstances, supplementary iron may be of great value in controlling anaemia in groups at special risk.

Ferrous sulfate tablets, given in small doses under supervision for a few weeks at a time, and repeated after an interval, are effective, inexpensive and carry no risk. Alternatively, it may prove possible to increase dietary iron content by adding small quantities of an iron preparation to a basic food in general use in the community. This presents technical difficulties but is worth investigation. Another important approach is to encourage people to modify their diets so as to increase consumption of foods rich in iron and substances that enhance iron absorption and to reduce consumption of substances that impair iron absorption.

Sanitation

There are no important reservoir hosts for *A. duodenale* and *N. americanus* other than man, and all the hookworm eggs that perpetuate human infection enter the environment in human faeces. Universal safe disposal of faeces would eradicate hookworm infection and, in fact, has done so in several developed countries. Thus, improved sanitation is always an important goal in hookworm control, particularly in rural areas where indiscriminate defecation and the agricultural use of uncomposted human faeces pollute the soil.

Well designed, sanitary latrines are relatively expensive to build and may be a more sophisticated measure than is strictly necessary for the control of hookworm infection. However, as they also contribute to the control of other diseases, they may be a good investment if adequate resources exist both for their construction and for their subsequent maintenance. Maintenance of latrines has often proved to be a much greater problem than construction, leading to their abandonment and loss of the investment made. Much work has been done on the design of latrines that function with little or no need for water (6), but again the problem is less one of design and construction than of supervision, cleaning and maintenance.

Where, for one reason or another, it is not possible to provide a sufficient number of latrines to meet the needs of the community, hookworm transmission may be reduced by persuading people to defecate in places that are unfavourable for development of hookworm larvae or in a way that minimizes exposure to infective larvae. However, this 'sanitation without latrines' requires health education and is possible only where defecation habits can be discussed openly. The approach would probably prove most successful in south-east Asia, where such discussion is possible and where, in fact, local traditions already prescribe appropriate defecation behaviour. Traditional practices can be encouraged or discouraged, depending on the protection they provide from hookworm infection.

Both the time and the place of defecation are significant factors in hookworm transmission. In tropical areas, eggs in faeces will be killed rapidly by the high stool temperatures reached at midday on sunny days. Direct sunlight is unfavourable to larval development: faeces heat up quickly and both they and the soil surface dry out rapidly. Defecation is thus less dangerous in open, dry, fallow fields or other sun-baked areas than in shaded, moist areas. Where latrines are not available, the use of simple pits or trenches provides good hookworm control (although they may encourage flies to breed if left uncovered).

Individuals will be protected from exposure to hookworm infection if they squat over the edge of steep slopes (railway embankments, dikes of paddy fields, pond edges, etc.) to defecate. Similarly, the use of raised pedestals (bricks, logs, bamboo stubs or low horizontal tree trunks) as squatting places protects the feet from contact with infective larvae. The accumulation of faeces in heaps in such areas provides unfavourable conditions for the hatching and development of hookworm larvae. However, these methods afford no protection against other faecally borne diseases and may, in fact, exacerbate some (e.g. schistosomiasis).

To summarize, sanitation:

- reduces or interrupts transmission of hookworm infection
- prevents reinfection
- gradually reduces hookworm loads as the older worms die off
- is slow to take effect
- is costly unless adopted as a community effort
- has no immediate effect on hookworm anaemia unless combined with iron and anthelminthic treatment, but
- is essential for any lasting benefit.

Health education

Regardless of the epidemiological situation, the sections of the population most affected, the combination and phasing of control measures chosen and the size of the programme, health education has an essential role in the control of hookworm.

In the preparatory stages of a control programme, health education plays a large part in securing the support of the influential groups in the community (village chiefs, local politicians, religious leaders, schoolteachers, women's organizations, employers of agricultural workers and others).

During the implementation phase, which may extend over several years, there are two main purposes to health education. The first is to inform all sections of the community about hookworm anaemia, its effect on their health and prosperity, how to avoid it and how to control it. This should be carried out on a continuing basis and should include special instruction of village health workers and schoolteachers, who can then instruct others and ensure such continuity.

In this regard, health education:

- teaches people how they acquire the disease
- shows them how to avoid becoming infected
- persuades them to change their defecation behaviour
- explains how to reduce or avoid contact with infected soil
- advises against the use of uncomposted human manure
- proposes acceptable alternatives to harmful practices
- teaches people how to use sanitation facilities properly
- encourages them to wear shoes

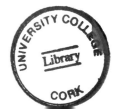

- shows them how to increase the iron content of their diet and promote its absorption.

The second, and usually more difficult, task is to keep the community informed of progress and to encourage participation in and compliance with control measures after the initial enthusiasm and novelty have declined.

6. Assessing the situation

Awareness that a health problem exists

At all levels of the health service, patients tend to present with the symptoms and signs of anaemia, rather than complaining of the hookworm infection that may be the underlying cause.

If anaemia is common in an area, it will probably already have been recognized as a health problem, although its nature and epidemiology may not be fully understood. Even where health services are limited and laboratory facilities rudimentary, it will often be common knowledge that many people have the symptoms of anaemia, and some indication of the extent of the problem may be available from health staff.

This is usually not the case with hookworm infection, however, which may remain undetected or unsuspected as a cause of anaemia, in spite of the sporadic observation of hookworm eggs in stool samples.

Once it is known that anaemia presents a significant problem and that hookworm infection may be responsible, the steps outlined below will provide the basis for developing a programme for prevention and control in the community concerned.

In the tropics and subtropics:
- **where anaemia is common**
  - **— look for hookworm infection**
- **where hookworm infection is common**
  - **— look for anaemia**

Informing others and securing their help

Investigation of anaemia and hookworm infection may require the help of many people both within and outside the health sector, while the planning and implementation of control programmes may call for policy decisions by government and the formal involvement of various ministries. It is therefore important to ensure that all concerned are adequately informed at an early stage, and to seek their collaboration and the help of their staff in providing access to the records and facilities under their control. At the same time, an undertaking should be given to keep them informed of progress and to involve them in decisions about eventual control measures. To achieve this, and to avoid possible difficulties and misunderstandings, it will be necessary to hold coordination meetings at various administrative levels and with different community groups and organizations.

Collection and review of available data

At national or state level, annual reports of government health departments or public health laboratories may give a good indication of the extent of anaemia and hookworm infection in the population as a whole, the areas of greatest prevalence, and the groups most affected. Similarly, reports of occupational, school, and maternal and child health services may be sufficient to identify those at special risk, while reports of routine stool examinations or of special surveys by government laboratories may give an indication of hookworm prevalence in different parts of the country. Estimates of dietary iron and data on the general quality of the diet and the consumption of iron-rich foods and of substances that enhance or impair iron absorption may be available from the appropriate sections of ministries of health and agriculture.

Data may also be available from special studies made by environmental health services, medical schools, schools of public health, or other university institutions. The ministry of labour may be a source of useful information concerning the occupations in which hookworm infection is a particular health risk.

Health staff at provincial, regional or district level may already have fairly clear knowledge of the extent of hookworm infection and anaemia, of the importance of each and of the relationship between them. They may have found that most anaemic patients respond to treatment with iron; or that, if such treatment is stopped, patients soon become anaemic again; or that in pregnancy folic acid is also needed; or that anaemia does not generally respond well to iron and that causes other than simple iron deficiency must be sought.

Clinical and laboratory records from health centres or hospitals serving the area may provide confirmation of these observations and be able to supply data on prevalence, severity and types of anaemia and the case load they represent.

Such information, collected at all levels of health services and carefully reviewed, may allow a general appraisal of the public health situation with respect to anaemia and hookworm infection. However, hospital and health centre patients are a self-selected group and not necessarily representative of the population from which they come. Health statistics commonly supply only numbers and sex distribution of cases, with little indication of the types of anaemia; most cases are collectively described as "other specified and unspecified anaemias". It is therefore essential to supplement information of this type with special haematological and parasitological surveys.

Before surveys are planned, it is important to establish whether similar exercises have already been carried out and whether results were published. Earlier surveys may contain valuable information that perhaps needs only to be updated.

General survey

Properly planned and carried out, a combined hookworm and anaemia survey will:

- measure the prevalence, intensity and distribution of hookworm infection and the prevalence, severity and distribution of anaemia in the community;

- show whether the anaemia is mainly of the iron deficiency type and provide an estimate of the proportions of *A. duodenale* and *N. americanus* present in those affected; and

- establish a baseline against which the results of prevention and control measures may be assessed.

Generally speaking, it is advisable to limit the coverage of the initial surveys to a few communities at a time. This allows many of the practical problems commonly encountered in such work to be identified and overcome and will greatly facilitate subsequent larger-scale surveys.

The sequence of surveys and the information to be derived from them are summarized in Fig. 8. Stool and haemoglobin surveys should be made concurrently on the same sample of the community, so as to maximize the value of the information obtained; this also applies to the more detailed parasitological and haematological investigations to be made on subsamples.

Techniques for use in hookworm and anaemia surveys are described in Annexes 1 and 2 respectively. The importance of taking truly representative samples is evident, if valid conclusions are to be drawn and major

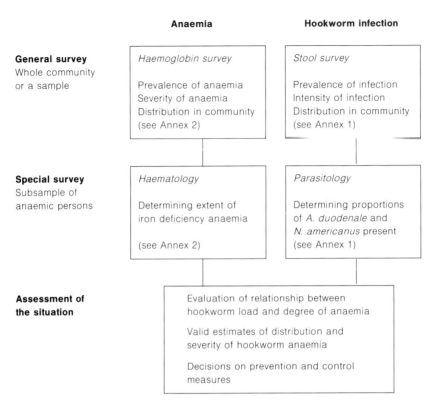

Fig. 8. Sequence of anaemia and hookworm surveys

sources of bias and error avoided. Suitable methods for sampling are described in Annex 3.

The results of haemoglobin and stool surveys may conveniently be recorded on a registration form, as shown in Table 9, which indicates at a glance whether certain households or families are more affected than others. This, in itself, may give important clues to the principal means by which hookworm infection is transmitted and the cause of anaemia in the area.

It is generally accepted that, at a given altitude and in the absence of disease or inherited abnormality, the normal range of haemoglobin levels varies with age, sex and pregnancy but not with ethnic differences or climate. Normal haemoglobin values and the levels below which anaemia may be presumed to exist are shown in Table 10.

> **In the tropics and subtropics there is no
> reason to accept low haemoglobin levels as "normal"—
> if they are low there is a cause**

Table 9. Anaemia and hookworm survey registration form

Date:

Village:

Examined by:

District:

Serial no.	Household no.	Family and given name	Age	Sex M F[a]		Occupation[b]	Haemoglobin g/litre	Hookworm eggs/g faeces

[a] Women—indicate P if pregnant, L if lactating.
[b] Occupation—indicate type: agriculture, plantation, mines, tunnel works, etc.

Table 10. Normal haemoglobin values and indicators of anaemia

Group	Normal mean values of Hb (in g/litre)	Indicators of anaemia[a] (Hb in g/litre)
Men	158	< 130
Women	139	< 120
Pregnant women		< 110
Children		
12 months	116	
2 years	117	< 110
4 years	126	
6 years	127	
8 years	129	
10 years	130	< 120
12 years	134	

[a] Haemoglobin levels below which anaemia may be presumed to exist.

From the basic register of people included in the survey (Table 9), further tables may be prepared showing the relation between haemoglobin levels and hookworm egg counts for each section of the community (men, women, children).

For this purpose, it is helpful to group individual haemoglobin levels and hookworm egg counts by intervals. Although these groups are arbitrary they facilitate statistical analysis, examination of the relationship between haemoglobin levels and hookworm egg counts and the assessment of changes over time.

The following intervals are convenient and appropriate for use in surveys and have been used in Tables 11 and 12:

Haemoglobin (g/litre): < 30   30–59   60–89   90–119   ≥ 120
Hookworm egg counts (eggs/g of faeces):   0   < 1 000   1 000–2 999   3 000–9 999   ≥ 10 000

Table 11 serves as an example of both a tally sheet and a summary table for a given group. At this stage of the analysis, it is important to keep separate the findings for each group or section of the community, so that differences in prevalence, intensity of infection and haemoglobin levels between groups (children under 5 years, children of 5–14 years, men, women, pregnant women, etc.) may easily be recognized. Later, if no significant differences are found, a composite table may be prepared relating to the community as a whole.

Table 11. Example of a tally sheet for analysis of survey data

Date: _____   Examined by: _____

Village: _____   District: _____

Population group: _____

Haemoglobin g/litre	Hookworm eggs/g faeces					Subtotal
	0	< 1000	1000–2999	3000–9999	⩾ 10 000	
< 30						—
30–59						—
60–89		/	1 ///	3 /	1	5
90–119	LHT // 7	LHT /// 8	LHT // 7	// 2		24
⩾ 120	LHT // 7	LHT / 6				13
Total	14	15	10	3	—	42

Computerization of survey data may greatly facilitate analysis and assessment of the relationship between intensity of hookworm infection and the degree of anaemia.

Special survey

A subsample of those included in the general haemoglobin and stool survey should be selected for more detailed studies to determine the extent of iron deficiency anaemia (see Annex 2) and the proportions of *A. duodenale* and *N. americanus* present (see Annex 1).

This special survey should be representative of the different sections of the population (men, women, pregnant or lactating women, children). It should also be selective in that those chosen should be frankly anaemic, so that the results of the examinations made may be unequivocal. Any anti-anaemic or anthelminthic treatment received in the preceding six months should be noted, as it may affect the blood findings and the hookworm load.

People with a haemoglobin level of less than 60 g/litre would be suitable subjects for survey. If there are not enough people available with haemoglobin levels this low, the upper limit may be raised to 70 or 80 g/litre or to 90 g/litre, depending on circumstances.

The basic question to be addressed is whether the pattern of anaemia is predominantly one of iron deficiency; in most cases, relatively simple investigations will provide an answer. In general, a haemoglobin estimation, a packed cell volume, and examination of a stained blood film (all of which can be done on capillary blood) and subsequent calculation of the mean corpuscular haemoglobin concentration (MCHC) will show whether anaemia is of the iron deficiency type (hypochromic microcytic with a low MCHC) or has other characteristics. (See Annex 2.)

However, as the etiology of iron deficiency anaemia in the tropics and subtropics is often multifactorial, the results of routine blood examination may not always be conclusive. Where there is doubt, examination of stained bone marrow smears from a subsample (e.g. hospitalized patients with anaemia) will show whether erythropoiesis is normoblastic or megaloblastic, and, stained for iron, whether iron stores are present.

If adequate reference laboratory facilities are available and easily accessible, the iron status of the community may be assessed, using three biochemical measurements—plasma iron and total iron-binding capacity, which reflect iron availability to the tissues, and serum ferritin which is useful in detecting depletion of iron stores. However, since such facilities are not commonly available, it may be preferable to proceed directly to a therapeutic trial with iron, which will demonstrate conclusively, to health staff and the community alike, whether most cases of anaemia respond to iron treatment.

Examining survey data

Setting out the results of the haemoglobin and hookworm surveys for each population group as indicated in Table 11 shows clearly:

- the range of haemoglobin levels and hookworm egg counts in each group;
- whether low haemoglobin levels and moderate or high hookworm egg counts are common in any particular group; and
- whether those with low haemoglobin levels tend to have high hookworm egg counts (and vice versa) or whether there is no apparent correlation.

The examples given in Tables 12 and 13 illustrate the presentation of survey data. In this case, assuming that the 100 people surveyed constituted an adequate and representative sample of the population under study, the following observations may be made:

- *Anaemia*
  - 65% of those surveyed had a haemoglobin level below 120 g/litre; anaemia was therefore common;

Table 12. Haemoglobin levels and hookworm egg counts (examples from a survey)

Haemoglobin g/litre	Hookworm eggs/g faeces					Subtotal	
	0	⩽ 1000	1000–2999	3000–9999	⩾ 10 000	Number	%
Men							
< 30	—	—	—	—	—	—	
30–59	—	—	—	—	—	—	
60–89	—	—	—	5	—	5 ⎫	48%
90–119	—	3	3	5	—	11 ⎬	
⩾ 120	4	10	2	1	—	17	52%
Subtotal	4	13	5	11	—	33	
Women							
< 30	—	—	—	—	—	—	
30–59	—	—	—	—	—	—	
60–89	—	—	2	7	—	9 ⎫	80%
90–119	—	7	4	—	—	11 ⎬	
⩾ 120	2	3	—	—	—	5	20%
Subtotal	2	10	6	7	—	25	
Children under 15 yrs							
< 30	—	—	—	—	—	—	
30–59	—	—	—	—	—	—	
60–89	—	1	3	1	—	5 ⎫	69%
90–119	7	8	7	2	—	24 ⎬	
⩾ 120	7	6	—	—	—	13	31%
Subtotal	14	15	10	3	—	42	
All							
< 30	—	—	—	—	—	—	
30–59	—	—	—	—	—	—	
60–89	—	1	5	13	—	19 ⎫	65%
90–119	7	18	14	7	—	46 ⎬	
⩾ 120	13	19	2	1	—	35	35%
Total	20	38	21	21	—	100	
	20%	38%	21%	21%	—		100%

— all groups were affected: men 48%, women 80%, children 69% (note: using a haemoglobin level of 120 g/litre as an indicator underestimates anaemia in men and may overestimate it in children, depending on their age);

Table 13. Falling haemoglobin levels and rising egg counts
(grouped data from Table 12)

Haemoglobin g/litre	Hookworm eggs/g faeces < 1000	⩾ 1000	Subtotal
60–89	1	18	19
90–119	25	21	46
⩾ 120	32	3	35
Total	58	42	100

– severe anaemia (haemoglobin levels below 60 g/litre) was not found in any group; and

– haemoglobin levels above 120 g/litre were more common in men (52%) than in women (20%) and children (31%), but the differences were not statistically significant for the numbers involved ($P > 0.05$).

● *Hookworm*
  – 20% of those surveyed were not infected;
    80% were infected with hookworms;
  – 38% had fewer than 1000 eggs/g of faeces;
    21% had 1000 or more but fewer than 3000 eggs/g of faeces;
    21% had 3000 or more eggs/g of faeces;
  – higher levels of 10 000 or more eggs/g of faeces were not found;
  – men and women were infected with equal frequency and intensity; and
  – children appeared to be less often infected and to have lighter worm loads than adults.

● *Anaemia and hookworm infection*
  – low haemoglobin levels (less than 90 g/litre) were not found in those without hookworm infection;
  – haemoglobin levels of 120 g/litre and above were uncommon in those with hookworm egg counts of 1000 eggs/g of faeces or more;
  – the proportion of people with mild and moderate degrees of anaemia increased as hookworm egg counts rose; and
  – in the sample surveyed, a level of 1000 hookworm eggs/g of faeces appeared to be the dividing line above which anaemia increased in prevalence (see Table 13).

Analysing the results of haemoglobin and hookworm surveys in this way provides most of the information needed to define the extent, distribution and severity of anaemia and hookworm infection in a population.

Table 14. Main patterns in hookworm anaemia and infection

Anaemia	Hookworm infection
Mild to moderate anaemia common Few serious cases	Generally light infections
No particular group affected	No particular group affected
Severe anaemia common but mainly in certain groups	Infection common but greater intensity in certain groups
Severe anaemia common in all sections of the community	Infections of moderate or high intensity common in all sections of the community

One of three main patterns is likely to emerge; these are summarized in Table 14. Complemented by the special subsample surveys on the predominant type of anaemia and the proportions of *A. duodenale* and *N. americanus*, these data provide the basis for deciding whether hookworm anaemia is a significant health problem in an area and, if so, what should be the main features of a control programme.

7. Practical prevention and control

Programme approaches

The three main patterns of hookworm anaemia—already summarized in Table 14—are as follows:

- *Mild to moderate hookworm anaemia*
  Many people in the survey may be found to have haemoglobin values somewhat below normal, but marked or severe anaemia is uncommon. Similarly, hookworm infection may be widespread but egg counts are generally low. This situation can be dealt with by standard case management through primary health care, for the few who are severely anaemic, and by health and nutrition education and promotion of sanitation, which will lead to a gradual reduction in prevalence.

- *Severe hookworm anaemia in certain groups*
  Severe anaemia may be common among certain groups in the community yet relatively rare in others. Groups at risk include women of childbearing age, agricultural workers, plantation labourers, and others whose habits or occupations expose them to the risk of acquiring more intense hookworm infections than the rest of the population. In addition to standard case management, these groups require targeted, twice-yearly anthelminthic treatment to reduce hookworm loads, plus supplementary iron therapy to control anaemia. Some groups may also require special sanitation measures at their place of work.

- *Severe widespread hookworm anaemia*
  Where moderate to severe iron deficiency anaemia is widespread and affects all sections of the community (though possibly some more than others), the only practical approach may be to use mass treatment with iron supplements and an anthelminthic. This may mean that some receive treatment who do not need it, but the severity of the situation may justify the short-term expense until longer-term control measures can be instituted.

Table 15. Programme components for prevention and control of hookworm anaemia

Survey findings	Mass treatment	Targeted treatment	Standard treatment	Health education	Promotion of sanitation
Mild hookworm anaemia			■	■	■
Severe hookworm anaemia, only certain groups affected		■	■	■	■
Severe hookworm anaemia widespread in community	■		■	■	■

Management of hookworm anaemia following these three basic patterns is summarized in Table 15. Primary health care (with standard treatment), health and nutrition education, and the promotion of sanitation are essential in each case. Health education and the promotion of sanitation are beyond the scope of this manual and are not discussed further, but reference may be made to the report of the WHO Expert Committee on the Prevention and Control of Intestinal Parasitic Infections (*3*).

Control of hookworm anaemia in primary health care

At the primary health care level, treatment of the moderate to severe iron deficiency anaemia caused by hookworm infection (and prevention of resulting morbidity and mortality) is relatively easy. Programmes with this particular objective should always be integrated with any more general measures already in operation for the control of anaemia.

With appropriate instruction and supervision, the village health worker, midwife, leader or schoolteacher can be relied upon to:

- recognize moderate to severe anaemia;
- watch for new cases occurring in the community;
- administer oral iron therapy to those with anaemia;
- keep a register of people receiving treatment;

49

- administer an anthelminthic, if authorized to do so;
- refer to the nearest health post or treatment centre those who are seriously ill or who have not improved after 3–4 weeks' treatment with oral iron; and
- organize the routine oral administration of iron to women throughout pregnancy and lactation and to any other groups at special risk (combining this with a course of antimalarial treatment in malaria-endemic areas).

Thus, provided that the nature of the hookworm anaemia problem has been recognized, effective control can be achieved at village level with a minimum of resources. Given competent overall supervision and adequate supplies, this type of control at primary health care level can be extended to cover large areas. Although it will have little impact on the prevalence of hookworm infection in a community, it will keep iron deficiency anaemia under control until longer-term measures have time to take effect.

Treatment of hookworm anaemia

Iron deficiency anaemia caused by hookworm infection responds rapidly to treatment with oral iron preparations, even in patients who are profoundly anaemic. Injectable iron may be used in special cases where supervised oral treatment cannot be ensured, but is rarely necessary therapeutically.

After the start of iron treatment, a reticulocyte response may be seen in about 8 days. The patient begins to feel better and an improvement in clinical status and the haemoglobin level is usually noted by the third week. The haemoglobin rises by an average of 10 g/litre per week until normal levels are reached. This improvement occurs even without anthelminthic treatment but, if the hookworm load is not reduced, the haemoglobin level will start to fall again when iron therapy is discontinued. An anthelminthic should therefore be given early in the treatment of hookworm anaemia. In clinical management, any patient who requires iron therapy for hookworm anaemia also needs an anthelminthic.

Standard treatment in hookworm anaemia is summarized in Table 16.

In some areas where nutritional deficiencies are common, folic acid deficiency may coexist with, and be masked by, iron deficiency anaemia, revealing itself only in the failure of an anaemic patient to respond promptly and fully to iron treatment. In other cases, a blood smear may show a dimorphic picture with hypochromia, microcytosis and macrocytosis (which may indicate coexistent megaloblastic anaemia).

Table 16. Standard treatment in hookworm anaemia

Iron deficiency anaemia	Hookworm infection

Oral ferrous sulfate (200 mg tablet[a])
For adults:[b]
− 1 tablet 3 times daily for 2 months
  followed by
− 1 tablet daily for 4 months
	Anthelminthics
	At the start and at the end of iron
	treatment:[c]
	albendazole:
	− 400 mg in a single dose
	or
	mebendazole:
	− 500 mg in a single dose
	  or
	− 200 mg daily for 3 days

[a]One 200-mg tablet of ferrous sulfate contains 60 mg elemental iron.
[b]For children, use a smaller dose or other suitable preparation.
[c]In pregnancy, delay anthelminthic treatment until after delivery.

Patients with megaloblastic anaemia may look and feel much more ill than those with simple iron deficiency anaemia and may have marked anorexia. Two to three days after the start of treatment with folic acid, they may experience a dramatic return of appetite and a feeling of well-being—a rapid clinical (though not haematological) improvement that is not seen in patients treated with iron alone.

Combined deficiency of iron and folic acid is not uncommon in pregnancy and may be prevented by using tablets containing 60 mg iron and 200 μg folic acid as a nutritional supplement.

Where malaria is endemic, standard case management of hookworm anaemia may need to be supplemented by antimalarial treatment. In some parts of the world, thalassaemia is a common cause of hypochromic microcytic anaemia: this does not respond to iron therapy, which is contraindicated.

Treatment of hookworm infection

The choice of an anthelminthic for hookworm infection will depend on a number of factors and must be made on the basis of local considerations, including availability, cost, safety, efficacy, local experience, and whether treatment is on an individual or group basis.

Nowadays, hookworm infection is treated with anthelminthics such as albendazole, mebendazole, levamisole and pyrantel (dosages and chief characteristics are summarized in Table 17). These are broad-spectrum anthelminthics which are also effective against *Ascaris* species. Albendazole and mebendazole are highly effective and equally so against

Table 17. Recommended anthelminthics for hookworm infection

	Albendazole	Mebendazole	Levamisole	Pyrantel
Single dose	400 mg (all ages above 2 years)	500 mg	50–150 mg (3 mg/kg body wt)	—
		or		
Divided doses	—	100 mg twice daily for 3 days	—	10 mg/kg body wt (max. 1 g) daily for 3 days
Efficacy	+ + +	+ + +	+ +	+ +
Species sensitivity	A. duodenale = N. americanus		A. duodenale	N. americanus
Side-effects	Rare and mild gastrointestinal disturbances		Slight and transient gastrointestinal disturbances, headache and dizziness	
Contraindications	Age less than 2 years, or in pregnancy		Age less than 1 year, or in kidney disease or severe liver dysfunction	
Broad-spectrum, effective against:	Most nematode infections but less effective against Trichuris and Strongyloides stercoralis		Many nematode infections except Trichuris	

A. duodenale and *N. americanus*. This may be important in areas where *N. americanus* is the dominant species, since it has been reported as being less susceptible than *A. duodenale* to treatment with levamisole or pyrantel.

In light infections, a single annual treatment with an anthelminthic is sufficient, but in heavy infections a second treatment after 6 months is usually necessary. For individual patients, treatment spread over 3 days may offer some advantage, but single-dose treatment is essential for large-scale anthelminthic programmes.

Certain anthelminthics that were once very widely used and that are still employed in some places can no longer be recommended. They include tetrachlorethylene which, although the cheapest, has toxic effects and is contraindicated in ascariasis, bephenium which is relatively costly and unpleasant and should not be used in severe anaemia, in seriously ill children, during pregnancy or in patients with liver disease, and bitoscanate which has toxic effects.

The timing of targeted or mass anthelminthic treatment may be important in areas where transmission is seasonal. Two rounds of treatment, one at the end of the dry season and one at the end of the rainy season, should give the best results.

Implementation through other programmes

Epidemiological assessment, monitoring and evaluation should be under the control of the relevant department of the ministry of health. Actual prevention and control measures, however, should generally be implemented through other major programmes, such as community development, local government, women's organizations, maternal and child health, school and occupational health services, diarrhoeal disease control, water supply and sanitation, health education, or primary health care services, health centres and hospitals. The list is neither exhaustive nor in any order of priority, but it illustrates the importance of consulting all concerned, even at the early planning and investigative stages of a programme.

In effect, prevention and control of hookworm anaemia will succeed only if discrete, vertical programmes are avoided. Adoption of these objectives, and of appropriate methods of implementation, by other established health or community development programmes represents the best chance of continuity and success. This approach also offers to the existing programmes the opportunity to enhance their own local reputation and acceptance by participating in activities that bring rapid and obvious benefits to the communities concerned.

The community approach

Since the investigation of hookworm anaemia has to be made at community level, prevention and control should be planned at the same level and designed for the particular local circumstances. However, a series of investigations in different communities, spread over a wider area, may lead to the conclusion that the problems of hookworm infection and anaemia are basically similar throughout, and a common approach would then be appropriate.

Prevention and control, like initial investigation of the problem, should start at the lowest level, and the programme should then be developed upwards from this foundation to district and provincial or higher levels, as necessary.

Such an approach ensures that each community is fully involved from the beginning in investigating its own hookworm anaemia problem, in choosing the most suitable measures for prevention and control, in finding at least some of the resources required and in playing an active part in control measures.

Community members may contribute in many ways, for example by enlisting further public support, by keeping records, by distributing iron tablets to schoolchildren and pregnant women, and by providing labour and materials for latrine construction and drainage.

Planning a control programme

Programme planning is essentially a matter of balancing the appropriate measures and desired results with the resources available. Where hookworm anaemia has been found to be a significant health problem in a community, it can be brought under control at relatively little cost, even where health services and facilities are very limited.

Joint planning

The first step in planning a control programme should be to bring together everyone who has or will be involved, and to:

- present the results of the survey;
- identify the implications of the survey for the health of the community;
- assess the priority that should be given to action on hookworm anaemia;
- discuss the options available for effective control;
- outline the sequence of events in a control programme and the roles and responsibilities of the individuals and institutions concerned; and
- obtain agreement on targets, timing, resources and supplies, standard case management, screening methods, referrals, reporting, and other components of a joint programme.

Several such planning meetings may be necessary, at village, district and provincial levels.

Supervision and technical guidance

Supervision must be arranged at each level to ensure the proper coordination of activities, training of staff, availability of drugs and supplies, quality control of laboratory work, monitoring of progress and evaluation at suitable intervals.

At district level, the district medical officer would probably be the most suitable person to oversee all aspects of the programme and to mobilize help from community organizations. Where there is no district medical officer, the district hospital superintendent might take on this role.

Where a programme extends over several districts, the provincial health officer (or equivalent) would have responsibility for general coordination, supervision and technical guidance in the areas of provision of drugs, supplies and equipment, design of special health education, nutrition and sanitation programmes to complement iron supplementation and anthelminthic treatment, reporting on programme activities, collection of data on morbidity related to hookworm anaemia, orientation and training of staff, and assessment of costs, efficacy, efficiency, difficulties, trends and prospects of the programme.

While decentralization is important in the control of hookworm anaemia, institutions at regional or national level may be of great value in giving specialized training, by serving as reference centres for parasitology or epidemiology, and by ensuring an adequate and continuing supply of iron (or iron/folic acid) preparations and anthelminthics.

Monitoring and evaluation

Monitoring and evaluation are based on the same principles and techniques as the haemoglobin and hookworm surveys already described and should preferably be carried out by people who have acquired experience in the initial baseline surveys. The first question to be answered is:

● Do the measures introduced actually work: have they resulted in a reduction in the prevalence and severity of hookworm anaemia?

In hookworm anaemia, haemoglobin levels rise rapidly in response to iron therapy; if iron has been given to those who need it, the answer to the above question should be clearly positive within 3 months of starting therapy. The mean haemoglobin level should have risen and the number of people found to be anaemic should have fallen.

A haemoglobin survey is therefore the best way of monitoring progress. If undertaken 3, 6 and 12 months after the start of the programme, and thereafter at 12-month intervals, it is a sensitive measure of whether iron has been received by those who need it, whether supplements have been given for long enough and whether anthelminthics have been given where indicated.

Reductions in hookworm prevalence and intensity take much longer to become stable, and stool surveys (which require more organization and laboratory work) can safely be delayed until there is reason to believe that health education and sanitation programmes have had time to take effect. A temporary reduction in prevalence after the use of anthelminthics may be misleading.

Complementary information for monitoring and evaluation would include data on the numbers of people treated with iron and/or anthelminthics in each section of the population, the number of latrines constructed, and any other relevant modifications of defecation behaviour, the use of human manure, dietary habits and cooking practices.

Monitoring and evaluation should not only measure the impact of the programme but should also follow the manner in which the programme is implemented, asking questions such as:

- How is the drug supply being maintained?
- What degree of coverage is being achieved?
- Are people taking the medicines being offered?
- Are staff working as they should?

A process evaluation of this type is essential to success.

The results of monitoring and evaluation should be used to review and, where necessary, to revise the programme, for example by switching from mass treatment to targeted treatment or from targeted treatment to control through primary health care initiatives.

References

1. WALSH, J. A. & WARREN, K. S. Selective primary health care: an interim strategy for disease control in developing countries. *New England journal of medicine*, **301**(18): 967–974 (1979).

2. PETERS, W. The relevance of parasitology to human welfare today. Medical aspects— comments and discussion II. *Symposia of the British Society for Parasitology*, **16**: 25–40 (1978).

3. WHO Technical Report Series, No. 749, 1987 (*Prevention and control of intestinal parasitic infections*: report of a WHO Expert Committee).

4. YOKOGAWA, M. The control of soil-transmitted helminthiases in Japan. Unpublished WHO Document HELM./WP/66.7 (1966). (Available from Division of Control of Tropical Diseases, Information and Documentation Service, World Health Organization, 1211 Geneva 27, Switzerland.)

5. BLOCH, M. Intestinal parasitism. The importance of its correct location. *Revista del Instituto de Investigaciones Medicas*, **7**(2): 120–127 (1978).

6. WIMBLAD, U. & KILAMA, W. *Sanitation without water*. London, Macmillan, 1985.

Selected further reading

ADDY, D. P. Happiness is: iron. *British medical journal*, **292**(6526): 969–970 (1986).

ANDERSON, R. M. & MAY, R. M. Population dynamics of human helminth infections: control by chemotherapy. *Nature*, **297**: 557–563 (1982).

BANWELL, J. G. & SCHAD, G. A. Hookworms. *Clinics of gastroenterology*, **7**: 129–156 (1978).

BOTHWELL, T. H. & CHARLTON, R. W. *Iron deficiency in women*. Washington, DC, International Nutritional Anemia Consultative Group, 1981.

CORT, W. W. ET AL. A study on reinfection after treatment with hookworm and *Ascaris* in two villages in Panama. *American journal of hygiene*, **10**: 614–625 (1929).

GILLES, H. M. ET AL. Hookworm infection and anemia: an epidemiological, clinical and laboratory study. *Quarterly journal of medicine*, **33**: 1–24 (1964).

GILLES, H. M. Selective primary health care: strategies for control of disease in the developing world. XVIII. Hookworm infection and anaemia. *Reviews of infectious diseases*, **7**(1): 111–118 (1985).

HILL, R. B. Hookworm reinfestation in sanitated and unsanitated areas. *Southern medical journal*, **18**: 665–668 (1925).

HOAGLAND, R. E. & SCHAD, G. A. *Necator americanus* and *Ancylostoma duodenale*: life history parameters and epidemiological implication of two sympatric hookworms of humans. *Experimental parasitology*, **44**(1): 36–49 (1978).

KNIGHT, R. & MERRETT, T. G. Hookworm infection in rural Gambia. *Annals of tropical medicine and parasitology*, **75**: 299–314 (1981).

KOCHAR, V. K. ET AL. Human factors in the regulation of hookworm populations. In: Grollig, F. X. & Haley, H. B., ed. *Medical anthropology*. The Hague, Mouton, 1976.

KOMIYA, Y. & YASURAOKA, K. The biology of hookworms. In: Morashita, K. et al., ed. *Progress of medical parasitology in Japan*, Vol. 2. Tokyo, Meguro Parasitological Museum, 1966.

MATSUSAKI, G. Hookworm disease and prevention. In: Morishita, K. et al., ed. *Progress of medical parasitology in Japan*, Vol. 2. Tokyo, Meguro Parasitological Museum, 1966.

MILLER, T. A. Hookworm infection in man. *Advances in parasitology*, **17**: 315–384 (1979).

MULLER, R. *Ancylostoma, Necator* and ancylostomiasis. In: Feachem, R. G. et al., ed. *Sanitation and disease. Health aspects of excreta and wastewater management.* Chichester, Wiley, 1983.

ROCHE, M. & LAYRISSE, M. The nature and causes of hookworm anaemia. *American journal of tropical medicine and hygiene*, **15**: 1029–1102 (1966).

SAWYER, W. A. Factors that influence the rate of increase of hookworm infection. *American journal of hygiene*, **5**: 790–817 (1925).

SCHAD, G. A. & BANWELL, J. G. Hookworms. In: Mahmoud, A. A. F. & Warren, K. S., ed. *Tropical and geographical medicine.* New York, McGraw Hill, 1984.

SCHAD, G. A. ET AL. Arrested development in human hookworm infections: an adaptation to a seasonally unfavourable external environment. *Science*, **180**: 502–504 (1973).

SCHAD, G. A. ET AL. Human ecology and the distribution and abundance of hookworm population. In: Cross, J., ed. *Human ecology of infectious diseases.* New York, Academic Press, 1983.

SCHAD, G. A. & ANDERSON, R. M. Predisposition to hookworm infection in humans. *Science*, **228**: 1537–1539 (1985).

SCOTT, J. A. & BARLOW, C. H. Limitations to control of helminth parasites in Egypt by means of treatment and sanitation. *American journal of hygiene*, **27**: 619–648 (1938).

TOPLEY, E. Testing degree of anaemia: methods for use in developing countries. *Tropical doctor*, **16**: 3–8 (1986).

WHO. *Bibliography of hookworm disease (ancylostomiasis) 1920– 1962.* Geneva, World Health Organization, 1965.

WHO Technical Report Series, No. 277, 1964 (*Soil-transmitted helminths*: report of a WHO Expert Committee on Helminthiases).

WHO Technical Report Series, No. 666, 1981 (*Intestinal protozoan and helminthic infections*: report of a WHO Scientific Group).

YANAGISAWA, T. The epidemiology of hookworm disease. In: Morashita, K. et al., ed. *Progress of medical parasitology in Japan*, Vol 2. Tokyo, Meguro Parasitological Museum, 1966.

The following detailed reports on iron deficiency anaemia have been published by the International Nutritional Anemia Consultative Group, Los Angeles:

Guidelines for the eradication of iron deficiency anemia, 1977.
Iron deficiency anemia in infancy and childhood, 1979. (Also available in French and Spanish.)
Iron deficiency in women, 1981. (Also available in French and Spanish.)
The effects of cereals and legumes on iron availability, 1982.
The design and analysis of iron supplementation field trials, 1984.
Measurement of iron status, 1985.

These publications may be obtained by writing to The Nutrition Foundation Inc., 1126 Sixteenth Street NW, Washington, DC 20036, USA, or to Nutrition, World Health Organization, 1211 Geneva 27, Switzerland. Single copies for individuals from developing countries will be sent without charge.

Techniques for hookworm surveys

Hookworm surveys should provide three levels of information concerning each of the various population groups under study—the prevalence of infection, the intensity of infection, and the species of hookworm present.

Prevalence should be determined by using both *direct thin smear* and *cellophane thick smear* examination of faeces in a random or representative sample of the population. These two techniques are the basis of any survey of intestinal parasitic infections.

Intensity of infection is determined by the same *cellophane thick smear* used for prevalence determination; the number of hookworm eggs in a measured quantity of faeces is counted.

The *species* of hookworm present may be found by recovering the adult hookworms passed after treatment with an anthelminthic and counting the numbers of *Ancylostoma duodenale* and *Necator americanus*, or by identification of filariform hookworm larvae obtained by culture of faeces. In a survey of hookworm infection, faecal culture should be performed in 10% of cases with hookworm eggs present.[1]

Recording of survey findings

An example of a suitable record form for use in stool surveys is given in Table A1-1. The table should be accompanied by a map of the area.

Direct thin smear faecal examination

The direct thin smear is a simple examination technique and requires minimal equipment. It is suitable for the recognition of some protozoan cysts and trophozoites as well as for helminth eggs and larvae.

In preparation, care should be taken to use the right proportions of faeces (about 2 mg) and diluting fluid, so that the coverslip does not float. Saline, light Lugol solution, MIF solution (merthiolate, iodine, formol), and eosin solution are all suitable for use as diluting fluids.

---

[1] Further information may be found in:
Manual of basic techniques for a health laboratory. Geneva, World Health Organization, 1980.
Basic laboratory methods in medical parasitology. Geneva, World Health Organization, 1991.

Table A1-1. Example of a record form for stool survey

Date: Examined by:

Village: District:

| Serial no. | Household no. | Family and given names | Age | Sex | | Occupation | Finding in faecal smears | | Other notes |
				M	F		Direct	Thick	
1	2	3	4	5		6	7	8	9

Instructions

Columns 1 and 2:   Enter serial number of person examined and number of house as shown on survey map of village.

Column 5:   For women, indicate P if pregnant, L if lactating.

Column 6:   Indicate type: agriculture, plantation, mines, tunnel works, etc.

Column 7 and 8:   Note all helminths or protozoa found, using the following abbreviations: H—hookworm, A—*Ascaris*, T—*Trichuris*, E—*Enterobius*, S—*Strongyloides*, Ts—*Trichostrongylus*, G—*Giardia*, Eh—*Entamœba histolytica*, Ec—*Entamoeba coli*. The actual number of eggs found, rather than the number per gram of faeces, should be recorded for H, A, T.

Column 9:   Note any special feature about faecal material, e.g. blood, mucus, liquid, etc.

The direct thin smear has the advantage over the cellophane thick smear technique that hookworm eggs do not disappear in a slide preparation after a period of time. It does, however, have certain disadvantages: examination may be difficult because of the faecal debris present; the result of examination may be negative when the concentration of eggs is low (e.g. less than 1 000 eggs per gram of faeces); the result is not acceptable as a quantitative measure, even though the number of eggs found reflects to a certain extent the intensity of infection.

Differentiation of hookworm eggs

A guide to the recognition of intestinal helminth eggs is given in Fig. A1-1. Eggs of *A. duodenale* and *N. americanus* are oval with rounded, slightly flattened poles, about 50–70 μm in size; each has a very thin colourless shell, which appears as a thin black line under low magnification. The content, usually grey, varies according to the maturity of the egg. In a fresh stool, hookworm eggs usually contain 4, 8 or 16 cells. After a few hours, a mass of small granular cells is apparent and, after 12 hours, the eggs may already contain a hookworm larva. In routine laboratory practice, the eggs of *A. duodenale* are not distinguished from those of *N. americanus*; there is, in fact, a difference in size between the eggs of the two species but this is rarely a practical approach to distinguishing between them.

Hookworm eggs must be distinguished from:

Ascaris eggs	– semi-decorticated, fertilized: shell larger, about 70 μm, much thicker, double-lined, with a single round granular mass inside; – semi-decorticated, unfertilized: shell much larger, 80–90 μm, thicker, double-lined, refractile granules inside an amorphous grey mass filling the shell.
Enterobius eggs	– asymmetric, oval, thin, colourless but double-lined shell, containing embryonating cells or larva, but rarely blastomer stage.
Strongyloides spp. eggs	– smaller, about 50 μm, shell very thin, always contains a thick rhabditiform larva, rarely found in faeces.
Trichostrongylus spp. eggs	– much larger, 80–90 μm, asymmetric, oval, one pole rounded and the other narrower, shell the same as in hookworm eggs, contain at least 20 embryonic cells; the larval stage develops quickly.

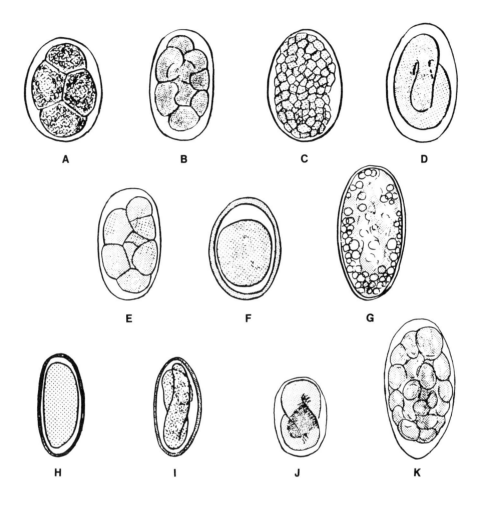

WHO 90448

A. *Ancylostoma duodenale* (early stage of development)
B. *A. duodenale* (a later stage—4, 8 or 16 cells)
C. *A. duodenale* (from stools a few hours old)
D. *A. duodenale* (from stools 12–48 hours old—larva developed)
E. *Necator americanus* (almost identical to *A. duodenale* in appearance)
F. *Ascaris lumbricoides* (semi-decorticated fertilized egg)
G. *A. lumbricoides* (semi-decorticated unfertilized egg)
H. *Enterobius vermicularis* (embryonating egg)
I. *E. vermicularis* (containing one larva)
J. *Strongyloides stercoralis* (egg very similar to *A. duodenale*)
K. *Trichostrongylus* sp.

Fig. A1-1. Morphology of eggs of common intestinal helminths

Cellophane thick smear faecal examination

The cellophane thick smear faecal examination technique was introduced in 1954 by Kato and Miura (1); it has proved to be a useful and efficient means of diagnosing intestinal helminthic infections, as well as *Schistosoma mansoni* and *S. japonicum* infections. Many modifications of the original technique have appeared since it was first published in English in 1966 (2).

The Kato and Katz modification of the quantitative cellophane thick smear is described below and illustrated in Fig. A1-2. The technique is relatively simple but must be performed carefully.

Materials

The following materials are required:

- Glass microscope slides—standard 25 × 75 mm slides are appropriate
- Flat-sided wooden applicator sticks—or similar devices made of plastic or other material
- Wettable cellophane—40 to 50 μm in thickness, in 22–25 mm × 30–35 mm strips.
- Glycerol solution, 50%—100 ml water, 100 ml glycerol
  Note: addition of 1 ml of 3% malachite green or 3% methylene blue solution, though not essential, makes the examination easier.
- Screen—either wire steel cloth (105 mesh stainless steel bolting cloth) or plastic screen (60 mesh per square inch or 250 μm mesh size). A stainless steel screen welded on to an oval steel ring with a handle is reusable.
- Template. Stainless steel, plastic or cardboard templates of varying diameters have been used (the size may depend on local requirements). This permits measurement of standard stool specimens and accurate egg counts.

The plastic spatula, plastic template and nylon screen in a commercially available Kato-Katz kit are shown in Fig. A1-2, plate 1. The first two items and the microscope slides may be reused. The nylon screen is disposable. A few kits may be ordered to provide standard reusable templates.[1]

---

[1] Information on commercially available Kato-Katz kits may be obtained from the Division of Control of Tropical Diseases, WHO, 1211 Geneva 27, Switzerland.

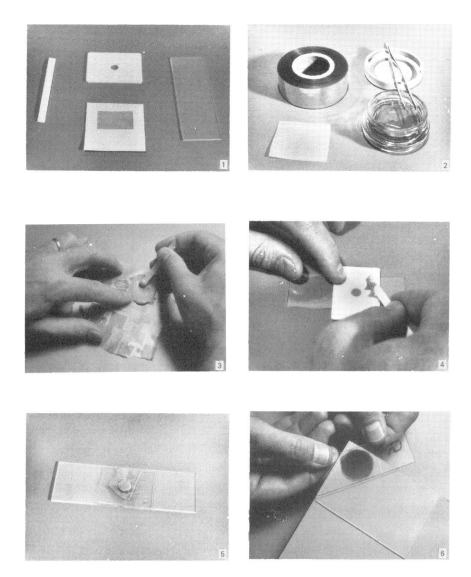

Fig. A1-2. Steps in using the cellophane faecal thick smear technique

The nylon screen and the cellophane required for the thick smear technique (see Fig. A1-2, plate 2) may be purchased in bulk. Cellophane is cut from the roll into 25–30 mm sections and placed in a wide-mouthed, flat-bottomed jar containing the 50% glycerol solution.

Procedure

(1) Soak the cellophane strips in the 50% glycerol solution for at least 24 hours before use.

(2) Transfer a small amount of faeces on to a piece of scrap paper (newspaper is satisfactory).

(3) Press the screen on top of the faecal sample.

(4) Hold the screen in place on the slide by fingertip pressure on one corner (see Fig. A1-2, plate 3). Force the faecal specimen through the screen, by means of a spatula, to separate faecal material with parasite eggs from particles of debris. (The spatula should be moved in a single outwards direction.)

(5) Place a template on a clean microscope slide so that it lies across the slide.

(6) Transfer a small amount of sieved faecal material into the hole of the template and carefully fill the hole. Level the faecal material with the applicator stick (see Fig. A1-2, plate 4).
Note: The original Kato-Katz template shown delivers about 42 mg of faeces, and the number of eggs observed is multiplied by 24 to obtain the number of eggs per gram of faeces. Other templates may have different volumes.

(7) Remove the template carefully so that all the faecal material is left on the slide with none sticking to the template.

(8) Cover the faecal sample on the slide with a glycerol-soaked cellophane strip (see Fig. A1-2, plate 5).

(9) If there is excess glycerol on the upper surface of the cellophane, wipe it off with a small piece of absorbent paper.

(10) Invert the microscope slide and press it against a piece of absorbent paper placed on a smooth flat surface (a piece of tile or flat polished stone can be used) to spread the sample evenly and remove excess fluid (see Fig. A1-2, plate 6).

(11) Lift up the slide, holding the piece of cellophane in place with a fingertip. After the slide is prepared, an additional drop of glycerol

may be placed on the cellophane and the edges of the cellophane pressed smooth to ensure conservation of the slide.

Reading the slides

An important limitation of the Kato-Katz technique is that, depending on local conditions of temperature and humidity, the delicate, thin-shelled hookworm eggs usually disappear soon after the thick smear has become clear enough for examination (because of the glycerol used). Eggs may have become invisible after 60 minutes. The slides should therefore be kept at room temperature and examined for hookworm eggs *as soon as possible* after preparation of the thick smear.

Under very hot and dry conditions, the clearing of slides and the disappearance of hookworm eggs may be slowed by placing the slides in a box or covering them to prevent evaporation.

Many different recommendations have been made regarding the reading time of the slides. *Ideally, every laboratory should review the reading procedure carefully to determine the optimal time, which may vary seasonally with the temperature and humidity.* In mounted cellophane thick smear preparations, hookworm eggs usually become invisible within a few hours.

The following correlations are useful in calculating the number of eggs per gram of faeces using the Kato-Katz technique (the multiplication factor is 24):

< 41 eggs/slide	< 1 000 eggs/g faeces
⩾ 42 eggs/slide	⩾ 1 000 eggs/g faeces
⩾ 125 eggs/slide	⩾ 3 000 eggs/g faeces
⩾ 417 eggs/slide	⩾ 10 000 eggs/g faeces

Egg counts may be influenced by a number of factors, including:

● number of hookworms—the more parasites, the fewer eggs produced per female worm;
● the age of hookworms—the very young and the old produce fewer eggs;
● seasonal variations in egg production;
● fluctuations in the weight of faeces produced daily; and
● quality of the faecal sample (e.g. hard or very liquid faeces).

All these factors should be borne in mind when making comparative studies.

Other techniques

Because of the technical limitations of the Kato-Katz technique for detection of hookworm eggs, a number of other techniques are in use for quantitative stool examination. These include Beaver's direct egg-count technique (*3, 4*), Stoll's dilution egg-count technique (*5*), and the McMaster technique using an original egg-counting slide (*6*).

Collection and identification of adult hookworms

In individual cases, or for research purposes, stools may be collected after adequate and appropriate anthelminthic treatment, emulsified with water in a bucket, and separated by successive decanting of the fluid and sieving of the residue.

The adult worms can be distinguished with a hand lens. Males measure 5–11 mm and females 9–13 mm in length and have dorsally curved anterior ends. *N. americanus* is more finely tapered anteriorly than *A. duodenale* and has a distinctly bent anterior tip. In contrast, the anterior part of *A. duodenale* tapers only slightly and its dorsal bend is less pronounced.

Examination under the microscope of the oral opening on the ventral surface of a hookworm permits a precise identification of the species. *A. duodenale* has two pairs of 'teeth', whereas *N. americanus* has two curved cutting plates. The species of male may also be distinguished by differences in the structure of the copulatory bursa. These features are shown in Fig. A1-3.

Faecal cultures for identification of hookworm larvae

The use of faecal cultures for routine detection of human hookworm infection was introduced more than 60 years ago, but not widely used for diagnosis until 1951 when Harada & Mori (*7*) introduced a simple test-tube culture method. The Harada-Mori type of culture, which consists of faeces smeared on a strip of filter-paper placed in a test-tube containing a small amount of water, has been used mostly for identifying the species of hookworm responsible for an infection. Sasa et al. (*8*) modified this technique, replacing the glass test-tubes by plastic sleeves (see Fig. A1-4).

The filariform larvae obtained after 7–10 days of faecal culture may be identified by microscopic examination, according to the method described below.

Materials

The following materials are required:

- Polyethylene tubing—30 mm wide and 0.05 mm thick, available as rolls 200 metres in length.
- Electric heating iron—for sealing the polyethylene tubes.
- Filter-paper strips—4 cm wide and 15 cm long.

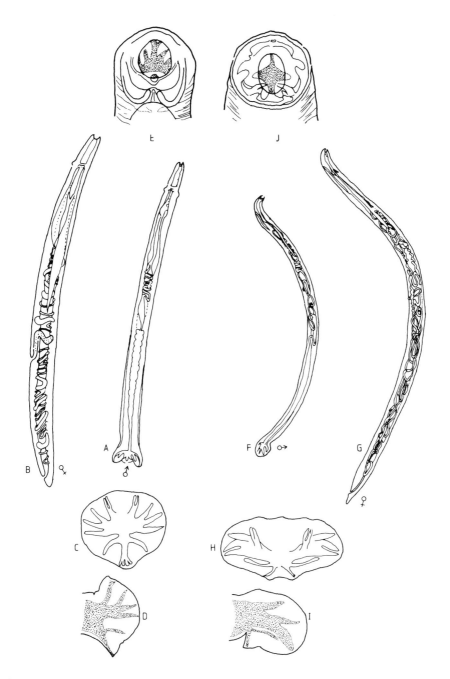

Fig. A1-3. Adult *Ancylostoma duodenale* and *Necator americanus*

A. duodenale A male, B female, C–D copulatory bursa, E buccal cavity
N. americanus F male, G female, H–I copulatory bursa, J buccal cavity
Redrawn from: BEAVER, P. C. & JUNG, R. C., ed. *Animal agents and vectors of human disease*, 5th ed. Philadelphia, Lea & Febiger, 1985.

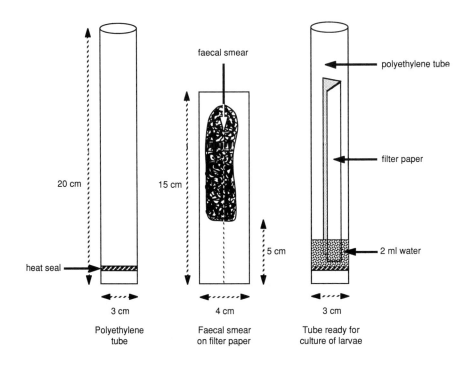

WHO 90446

Fig. A1-4. Polyethylene tube filter-paper culture method

Redrawn from: SASA, M. ET AL. A polyethylene-tube culture method for diagnosis of parasitic infections by hookworms and related nematodes. *Japanese journal of experimental medicine*, **35** (4): 277–289 (1965).

- Wooden applicators—about 15 cm long, for smearing faecal samples.
- Pasteur pipettes—for use with rubber bulbs or a 10 ml or 20 ml syringe.
- Forceps.
- Microscope slides and coverslips (18 mm × 18 mm).
- Beakers—containing heat-sterilized water.
- Stapler—for attaching polyethylene tubes together into bundles.
- Stereomicroscope—with low-power and high-power objectives or zoom lens.
- Compound microscope—with medium-power and high-power objectives (oil-immersion is unnecessary).
- Incubator—for use at 25 °C or 28 °C (usually unnecessary in tropical countries).
- Cigarette lighter or candle—for heating slides.
- Indelible pen—for marking the polyethylene tubes.
- Capillary pipettes—with rubber bulbs.

- Surgical gloves.
- Disinfectant.

Procedure

(1) Using scissors, cut the polyethylene tubing into pieces 20 cm long. Seal one end of each tube by using an electric iron (not above 45 °C). Add 2 ml of heat-sterilized water with a pipette or syringe.

(2) Fold the filter-paper strips in half lengthways and write the patient's name or number in pencil at the top.

(3) Take about 1 g of faeces with the wooden applicator and smear it on to the inner surface of a filter-paper strip, leaving about 5 cm unsmeared at one end of the paper and 2 cm at the other.

(4) Hold the smeared strip with forceps and insert it into a polyethylene tube, with the unsmeared 5-cm end at the bottom (see Fig. A1-4).

(5) With indelible ink, record the serial number or name of each patient on the polyethylene tube a few centimetres from its lower end.

(6) Collect 20 to 30 tubes prepared in this way, fold each tube at about 1 cm from the open end, and staple them together. The bundles of tubes can now be hung on a nail, a rod, or a string.

(7) Keep the tubes upright at 20–30 °C (ideally 28 °C) for 8–10 days.

(8) To examine the cultures, it is safer to wear surgical gloves to avoid infection by larvae if there is leakage of culture fluid. Hold a bundle of tubes with one hand and examine the bottom of each tube under low power with the stereomicroscope. Manipulate the tubes with the other hand, so that they can be examined by serial number in the right order. Most of the infective larvae are found at the base of the tube, but a few may be found in condensation water droplets on the tube wall or even near the top of the filter-paper strip.

(9) In order to identify the species, cut the tube and the unsmeared filter-paper about 4 cm from the bottom, collect the fluid and cut filter-paper in a watch-glass or Petri dish, examine them under the stereomicroscope, and pick up the larvae with a capillary pipette. Transfer the larvae, in a small drop of fluid, on to a slide, heat with a small flame directly under the glass until all the larvae stop moving. Never allow the fluid to boil. Identification may be made under the low-power lens of the compound microscope without using a coverslip, or under a high-power dry objective with a cover-slip. (Trained technicians can also differentiate the species of infective larvae in the tubes under the high-power magnification of the stereomicroscope.)

(10) After completion of the examination, the polyethylene tubes should be destroyed by burning and all other infective materials or equipment should be sterilized (e.g. by boiling).

Differentiation of nematode larvae in faecal cultures

Guidelines for routine practice in medical laboratories[1]

The presence of living larvae in the sediment can be detected using a hand lens (4 × or greater), a dissecting microscope or a special inverted microscope, and bright illumination from the side. If living larvae are observed, they should first be immobilized by immersing the bottom of the tube in water heated to 50–60 °C, or by adding a few millilitres of acetic acid (20 ml of glacial acetic acid in 80 ml of distilled water) to the suspension and mixing. If acetic acid is used the larvae should again be concentrated by centrifugation. The use of iodine for killing the larvae is not recommended since it tends to overstain them and this obscures their internal structures.

A drop or two of the sediment containing the killed larvae is transferred to a microscope slide (a wide slide is preferred) and an appropriate-sized coverslip added. If the examination is likely to be prolonged, the edges of the coverslip may be sealed with clear fingernail polish or melted paraffin to prevent evaporation.

The slide should first be examined under the low magnification (about 100 ×) of a compound microscope, with the light reduced by closing the stage diaphragm as much as possible so that the refractile larvae can easily be observed. When a larva is found, it should be examined under high power (about 400 ×) to observe the distinguishing features indicated in the key presented below. A calibrated ocular micrometer is required for determining measurements of larvae.

Since more than one type of larva may be present in a culture and the larvae of one species may be relatively few in number, all larvae recovered should be examined. The presence of larvae of different types can often be detected when the preparation is examined under low magnification.

Key for the identification of filariform nematode larvae in human coprocultures (see Fig. A1-5)

1a. Oesophagus about one-half length of body; body slender (14–17 μm), lacking cuticular sheath; tip of tail not pointed, appearing notched . . . . *Strongyloides* (*S. stercoralis* or *S. fuelleborni*)[2]

---

[1]Originally prepared by Dr M. D. Little, Department of Tropical Medicine, School of Public Health and Tropical Medicine, Tulane University, New Orleans, Louisiana, USA, and published in Annex 1 of *Intestinal protozoan and helminthic infections* (Report of a WHO Scientific Group). WHO Technical Report Series, No. 666, 1981.

[2]Filariform larvae of *Strongyloides stercoralis* and *S. fuelleborni* cannot easily be differentiated. Diagnosis must be made on the basis of stages occurring in fresh faeces (rhabditiform larvae in the case of *S. stercoralis*, and eggs containing a developing embryo in the case of *S. fuelleborni*) or on the morphology of free-living female worms from culture (prominent constriction of body behind vulva in *S. fuelleborni*; body not markedly constricted in *S. stercoralis*).

1b. Oesophagus about one-fourth of body length; cuticular sheath present; body thicker than 20 μm . . . . see 2

2a. Intestinal lumen straight . . . . see 3

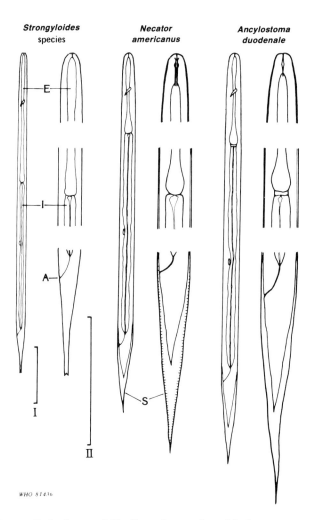

Fig. A1-5. Diagnostic features of filariform larvae found in human coprocultures

(A = anus, E = oesophagus, I = intestine, S = sheath. The scales represent 100 μm: I for intact larvae; II for portions of larvae).

Ternidens deminutus	Trichostrongylus species	Oesophagostomum species

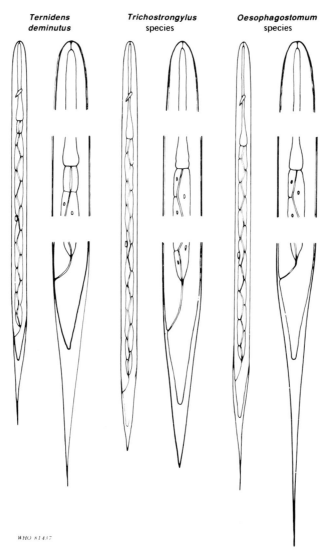

WHO 81437

Fig. A1-5 (continued)

2b. Intestinal lumen not straight but zigzagged . . . . see 4

3a. Body (not including sheath) about 500–600 μm long; tail (anus to tip)
less than 73 μm long (50–72 μm); intestine, at oesophagointestinal
junction, as wide as oesophageal bulb; buccal "spears" conspicuous,
parallel throughout length, about 15 μm long; conspicuous transverse
striations present on sheath in tail region . . . . . . *Necator americanus*

3b. Body (not including sheath) about 600–700 μm long; tail more than
73 μm long (75–94 μm); intestine, at oesophageintestinal junction,
narrower than oesophageal bulb; buccal "spears" inconspicuous,

about 10 μm long; transverse striations on sheath in tail region inconspicuous . . . . *Ancylostoma duodenale*

4a. Sheath relatively thin (thinner than cuticle of larva); pair of elongate sphincter cells present between oesophagus and first pair of intestinal cells; tip of larva's tail pointed; posterior end of sheath elongate, tapering to thread-like tip; body 630–730 μm long by 29–35 μm wide . . . . *Ternidens deminutus*

4b. Sheath relatively thick (thicker than cuticle of larva), no sphincter cells between oesophagus and intestine, tip of larva's tail rounded or blunt . . . . see 5

5a. Posterior end of sheath relatively short, not tapering to fine point (distance from tip of larva's tail to sheath less than distance from anus to tip of larva's tail) . . . . *Trichostrongylus* sp.

5b. Posterior end of sheath relatively long. tapering to a fine point (distance from tip of larva's tail to tip of sheath greater than distance from anus to tip of larva's tail) . . . . *Oesophagostomum* sp.

Note: Adult and larval stages of free-living nematodes (*Rhabditis* spp., *Pelodera* spp., *Rhabditoides* spp., etc.) may occur in cultures of faeces if contaminated with soil, and must be differentiated from larvae of the human parasites. It is possible that the first-stage larvae of *Angiostrongylus costaricensis* may occur in the faeces of some infected individuals and may appear in coprocultures. These larvae are 260–290 μm long and 14–15 μm wide, much smaller than any of the filariform larva mentioned in the above key.

References

1. KATO, K. & MIURA, M. Comparative examinations. *Japanese journal of parasitology*, **3**: 35 (1954).
2. KOMIYA, Y. & KOBAYASHI, A. Evaluation of Kato's thick smear technique with a cellophane cover for helminth eggs in faeces. *Japanese journal of medical science and biology*, **19**: 59–64 (1966).
3. BEAVER, P. C. Quantitative hookworm diagnosis by direct smear. *Journal of parasitology*, **35**: 125–135 (1949).
4. BEAVER, P. C. The standardization of faecal smears for estimating egg production and worm burden. *Journal of parasitology*, **36**: 451–456 (1950).
5. WHO Technical Report Series, No. 255, 1963 (*CCTA/WHO African conference on ancylostomiasis, Brazzaville, 22–29 August 1961*) (Annex 2).
6. THIENPOINT, D. ET AL. *Diagnosing helminthiasis through coproscopical examination.* Beerse, Janssen Research Foundation, 1979, pp. 40–41.
7. HARADA, Y. & MORI, O. [A simple method for the cultivation of hookworm larvae.] *Igaku to seibutsugaku*, **20**: 65–67 (1951) (in Japanese).
8. SASA, M. ET AL. A polyethylene-tube culture method for diagnosis of parasitic infections by hookworms and related nematodes. *Japanese journal of experimental medicine*, **35**(4): 277–289 (1965).

Techniques for hookworm anaemia surveys

Although hospital records and laboratory findings on anaemic patients may give an indication of the predominant type of anaemia in a particular area, this cannot be assumed. Hospital patients tend to have a higher prevalence of relatively unusual forms of anaemia and data relating to them may not reflect the situation in the general population. However, approaching the problem of anaemia on a community basis from the outset avoids this and other difficulties, since the possible causes of widespread anaemia in a community are few; in hospital patients, many possibilities may have to be taken into account. A community anaemia survey is therefore essential.

Because facilities, personnel, resources and time may be limited, it is important to obtain the maximum information from the survey so that valid general conclusions may be drawn for the community as a whole or for that section of it under investigation.

The haemoglobin surveys and subsequent blood examinations should answer the following questions:

- Is anaemia a problem in the area? If so:
  - is it mild or severe?
  - does it affect all sections of the community?
  - are some groups more affected than others?

- Is anaemia mainly hypochromic and microcytic? If so, is this true for all sections of the community?

- Is macrocytosis also a feature of some blood films? If so, is this due to a reticulocytosis or to coexistent megaloblastic anaemia?

Answers to these questions will provide the basis for public health action.

While the examinations required are simple, techniques must be meticulous at all stages if the results are to be reliable. It is therefore preferable for the survey to be self-sufficient, with its own field and laboratory technicians, equipment and, if necessary, transport so that the quality of the work may be assured and consistent. Several publications (e.g. *1, 2*) provide valuable guidance on techniques, interpretation and quality control.

Selection of people for examination

The haemoglobin survey should cover all people in a random or representative sample of the community selected for study (see Annex 3), whose faeces should also be examined for hookworm eggs.

From this sample, a subsample should be taken, consisting of all those anaemic persons with a haemoglobin level below a specified value, e.g. less than 60 g/litre. Depending on the numbers available, it may be necessary to raise this level to obtain sufficient subjects.

The following haematological examinations should be undertaken on this subsample to characterize the main types of anaemia present, the haemoglobin level being redetermined so that all tests are related to the same sample of blood:

– haemoglobin
– packed cell volume
– peripheral blood smear
– reticulocyte count
– thick blood film (where malaria is present in the area).

In certain cases or areas, it may also be necessary to examine a bone marrow smear to assess body iron status and to confirm suspected megaloblastic anaemia.

Haemoglobin estimation

The method used for haemoglobin estimation will depend on the equipment and facilities available (*3*), but the most reliable is the cyanmethaemoglobin method, using a filter photometer or spectrophotometer. This is the method of choice: a satisfactory standard is available and all forms of clinically significant haemoglobin can be measured. (Some suitable photometers can be operated either on mains electricity or on current from a motor vehicle battery.) Accuracy in measuring haemoglobin levels is essential where the mean level is to be calculated, but is less important where only a general indication of the prevalence of anaemia is required.

For field work, which may be performed under difficult conditions, other methods may be needed. The oxyhaemoglobin method, employing a photometer, is the simplest and quickest but has certain disadvantages.

A stable oxyhaemoglobin standard is not available and must therefore be prepared and checked against a cyanmethaemoglobin reference preparation, so that the photometer can be calibrated. The method does not measure all forms of haemoglobin, and the haemoglobin (HbO_2) solution fades rapidly and must be read within 6–8 hours.

Direct reading grey-wedge haemoglobinometers, which measure the absorption of light by oxyhaemoglobin in a thin layer of haemolysed blood, are battery-operated, based on visual comparison of optical density and convenient for field use. They require technical skill in use and careful cleaning of the chamber between samples if serious errors are to be avoided. The American Optical (AO) haemoglobinometer is accurate and has been used under tropical conditions for many years (see Fig. A2-1).

Other available methods cannot be recommended for survey work of this nature. The Talquist method, which compares the colour of a drop of blood on a piece of absorbent paper with a colour standard, has an error of up to 50%. The Sahli method is slow and laborious, with an error of up to 20%. The copper sulfate method is inconvenient, requires very accurate preparation of standard solutions and provides only an indication of whether haemoglobin is above or below certain selected fixed levels. This last may be used if better methods are not available but only for small-scale surveys: for large studies it is contraindicated.

Packed cell volume (PCV) determination[1]

Packed cell volume is determined using the micromethod, with a capillary tube of anticoagulated blood centrifuged for 5 minutes. The procedure is simple and reproducible, reliably indicates the degree of anaemia and often provides additional valuable information. In iron deficiency or inflammation, the supernatant plasma is pale; in megaloblastic or haemolytic anaemia, it has a deep yellow colour; and the greyish-white layer above the packed red cells may indicate high leukocyte or platelet counts. The plasma can be frozen and kept for subsequent serological examination.

Mean corpuscular haemoglobin concentration[1]

Mean corpuscular haemoglobin concentration may be calculated from the haemoglobin and the packed cell volume and gives an objective

---

[1] The traditional terms are used since they are likely to be more familiar to most readers than the recently introduced SI terms – erythrocyte volume fraction (for PCV) and mean erythrocyte haemoglobin concentration (for MCHC).

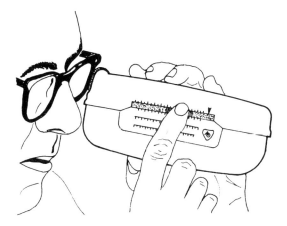

Fig. A2-1. Measuring haemoglobin with an AO haemoglobinometer

measurement of the degree of saturation of red blood cells with haemoglobin. The normal range is 320–370 g/litre and values below 320 g/litre are found in hypochromic microcytic anaemia. In marked iron deficiency anaemia, values of 160–240 g/litre are common.

Peripheral blood smear

A stained thin blood film, well prepared and carefully examined, is of great value. In iron deficiency anaemia, the typical findings in the red blood cells are:

- hypochromia – cells have a central pale area greater than half the cell diameter;
- microcytosis – cells are smaller than normal;
- anisocytosis – variations in cell size;
- poikilocytosis – variations in cell shape; a few target cells and elongated forms are present.

At haemoglobin levels below 90 g/litre, these signs become increasingly prominent.

In addition to iron deficiency anaemia of nutritional origin or caused by hookworms or chronic blood loss, a similar blood picture of hypochromia and microcytosis occurs in thalassaemia and haemoglobinopathies and in sideroblastic anaemia in which there is an inability to use iron properly. In mild degrees of anaemia, the blood picture in all these conditions may be indistinguishable.

A scheme for investigating patients with hypochromic microcytic anaemia is shown in Fig. A2-2. It is intended only as a guide and may require modification to suit local conditions or laboratory resources.

Laboratory test   **Interpretation**

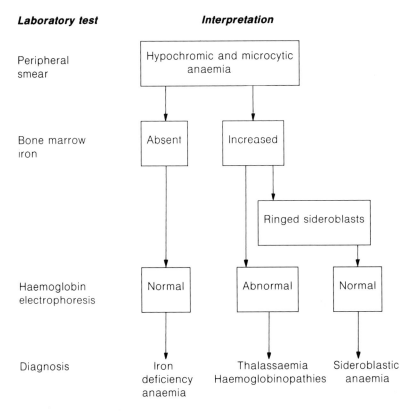

Fig. A2-2. Scheme for investigating patients with microcytic hypochromic anaemia

Where laboratory resources are limited, it is practical to make a tentative diagnosis of iron deficiency and to proceed to a closely supervised therapeutic trial with iron. A reticulocyte response and a rise in haemoglobin will confirm the diagnosis; if they do not occur, further investigations are indicated.

Where anaemia is widespread in a community, sideroblastic anaemia may be excluded, since it is a problem of individual patients only and not of groups. Thalassaemia and other haemoglobinopathies may have to be considered but, if there is no splenomegaly or reticulocytosis, are unlikely to be the cause of marked hypochromic microcytic anaemia. Absence of stainable iron in a bone marrow smear would confirm this view.

The presence of hypersegmented polymorphonuclear cells may be an indication of the coexistence of megaloblastic anaemia, which may become obvious only when the iron deficiency has been adequately treated with iron and the patient has failed to respond completely. In such a case, the original blood picture may be dimorphic, containing a mixture of hypochromic microcytic red blood cells and macrocytes. A bone marrow smear is indicated for final diagnosis.

Occasional large, bluish-staining red cells are likely to be reticulocytes and special staining for a reticulocyte count will show whether this is so.

Reticulocyte count

Normally, between 0.2% and 2.0% of red cells are reticulocytes, which are juvenile forms. Reticulocytosis is not a feature of chronic iron deficiency anaemia associated with hookworm infection, but it is found in haemolytic conditions — haemolytic anaemias, haemoglobinopathies and malaria — and in patients receiving effective treatment for anaemia.

Bone marrow smear

Where there is any doubt about the true nature of hypochromic microcytic anaemia or iron status in a community, a further subsample should be selected for bone marrow smears. Bone marrow aspiration can be done under field conditions, presents little risk, causes only slight discomfort and, with adequate explanation to the patient, is well accepted.

Stained for iron, a bone marrow smear provides a clear indication of whether or not hypochromic microcytic anaemia is due to iron deficiency. With ordinary staining, it will show the state of erythropoiesis and may reveal the presence of megaloblastic anaemia, due to folic acid and/or vitamin B_{12} deficiency, which often coexist with iron deficiency anaemia in the tropics and subtropics.

Red blood cell counts

Red blood cell counts using a haemocytometer are time-consuming and unreliable; they provide no extra useful information and have no place in a survey of hookworm anaemia.

Malaria parasites

In areas where malaria is endemic or where it is suspected, thick and thin blood films should be examined for malaria parasites.

Presentation of survey data

A simple and effective way of presenting data from haemoglobin surveys is to classify results by broad groups reflecting the degrees of anaemia found in different sections of the population surveyed, for example as in Table A2-1.

Table A2-1. Summary results of haemoglobin survey in a community

Group	Number in each group	Distribution of haemoglobin levels (g/litre) by class intervals									
		< 30		30–59		60–89		90–119		≥ 120	
		No.	%	No.	%	No.	%	No.	%	No.	%
Men											
Women											
Pregnant women											
Children: < 5 years 5 – 12 years											
Total											

These results may also be presented in the form of a histogram, which can be drawn quickly, requires no calculations and greatly facilitates an appraisal of the situation. Fig. A2-3, for example, shows the distribution of haemoglobin values of 200 adult men before and after 3 months' treatment with oral ferrous sulfate. The sharp reduction in the number of men with haemoglobin levels below 60 g/litre and the trend towards normal haemoglobin values are clearly shown in the histogram.

The extent and severity of anaemia are readily apparent from such histograms, comparisons between groups and assessment of change over time can easily be made and calculations are reduced to a minimum.

For community surveys in areas where anaemia is common, this method is preferable to the conventional calculation of the arithmetic mean and standard deviation, particularly as the distribution of haemoglobin levels is likely to be severely "skewed".

The findings of the haematological examinations made on subsamples of anaemic people covered in the haemoglobin survey may be summarized as in Tables A2-2 and A2-3. Similar tables may be prepared for reticulocytes and malaria parasites, and for bone marrow smears to show the type of erythropoiesis and the presence of stainable iron. For these groups it is useful to calculate the arithmetic mean and standard deviation, which facilitate analysis of the results of treatment.

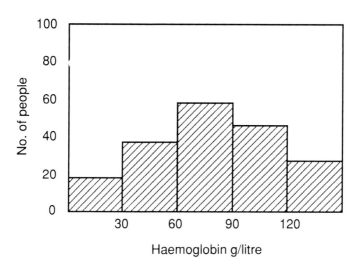

A. Before iron treatment

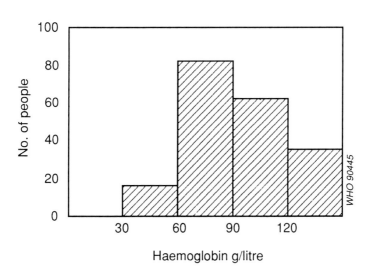

B. After iron treatment

Fig. A2-3. Haemoglobin levels of 200 adult men

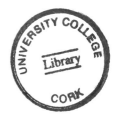

Table A2-2. Blood values of anaemic people

Group	Number in each group	Haemoglobin (g/litre)		PCV		MCHC (g/litre)					
		Mean	Range	Mean	Range	< 240		240–319		⩾ 320	
						No. %		No. %		No. %	
Men											
Women											
Pregnant women											
Children:											
< 5 years											
5–12 years											

Table A2-3. Peripheral blood slide findings in anaemic people

Group	Number in each group	Hypochromia No. %	Microcytosis No. %	Macrocytosis No. %	Anisocytosis No. %	Poikilocytosis No. %
Men						
Women						
Pregnant women						
Children:						
< 5 years						
5–12 years						
Total						

References

1. EVATT, B. L. ET AL. *Anemia – fundamental diagnostic hematology.* Atlanta, Centers for Disease Control, 1983.
2. *Manual of basic techniques for a health laboratory.* Geneva, World Health Organization, 1980.
3. TOPLEY, E. Testing degree of anaemia: methods for use in developing countries. *Tropical doctor,* **16**: 3–8 (1966).

Sample survey considerations

Scope of a survey

Surveys for the presence and intensity of hookworm infection and/or anaemia, like any similar health-directed surveys, provide opportunities for gathering data on the general status of the community. Since it is rarely possible to examine everyone in a population because it would take too long or cost too much or because insufficient personnel are available, a *sample* of homes or of individuals is selected and the information derived from examination of this sample is extrapolated to the larger community. Such surveys give reliable results only if the sample is representative of the population, if the sample is selected in an appropriate statistical manner, if cooperation of people can be assured and if the size of the sample is large enough to obtain estimates with the required degree of confidence. Considerable judgement is therefore essential in deciding the scope of a survey. On the one hand, it should not be complicated by the collection of data not strictly relevant to the problem under investigation. On the other hand, it should not be too restrictive and miss the opportunity of gaining a more penetrating insight into the health situation of the larger community.

These are matters to be decided in a local context and general guidance is difficult; as a basic principle, however, there should be no attempt to collect more information than resources allow or than can be properly analysed and evaluated.

Types of survey in hookworm infection

The study of hookworm infection or hookworm anaemia requires one of two types of survey – household or group – to assess the nature and extent of the problem.

Household surveys

Examination of all the members of a representative sample of the households in an area permits an estimation of the prevalence and severity of anaemia and of the intensity of hookworm infection for each section of the community by age, sex, occupation, economic status, special status (e.g. pregnancy), etc.

In an area where hookworm infection and anaemia are suspected, household surveys offer the optimum method of fully assessing the impact of infection on the local population and the factors determining its transmission. The plotting of survey results on a large-scale map may reveal the main sources of hookworm infection and the geographical distribution of those most severely affected. This may be of great value in deciding on the most appropriate strategy and tactics for control.

If there is some knowledge about the population in the area to be surveyed, a sampling scheme appropriate to the situation and the financial and logistic constraints can be selected, such as simple random sampling, stratified sampling or cluster sampling. The selected scheme may need to be carried out in one or two stages. Where there is little knowledge of the area or where the affected population is dispersed over a number of villages, it may be wise to select one small area of 200–300 people and examine everyone. In such a case, the problem of the correct choice of sampling procedure does not arise, but the prevalence and intensity rates obtained will give an indication of the range of values likely to be found in neighbouring villages. Such information is necessary in deciding on the best sampling frame and on the sample size.

Group surveys

Where it is known already that hookworm anaemia is a problem in specific sections of the population (e.g. in women or in a plantation labour force), surveys may concentrate on these particular sections, drawing representative samples from the groups to be examined.

Statistical guidance

The help of a statistician or epidemiologist should be obtained during the planning stage of a survey in order to obtain maximum benefit for the effort expended. Guidance may be needed to merge the results of small or limited surveys to give a reliable picture of the situation in a larger population. Extra time spent in planning is well repaid by the results of analysis. In 1985 WHO published a useful review of health surveys in general.[1]

---

[1] *World health statistics quarterly*, **38**(1): 1985.

Sample sizes for estimating prevalence

Surveys on hookworm infection or anaemia are carried out to determine the prevalence and intensity of the condition. The minimum sample size needed for a survey is dependent on the expected prevalence or the variation of the estimate of intensity; in principle the sample size can be determined for both. In practice, determination of sample size requirements is focused on the estimate of prevalence rather than intensity. For reliable estimations of the prevalence of hookworm infection or anaemia in a population, it is sufficient to select a sample such that the true rate for the population as a whole lies, with 95% confidence, within 5 percentage points of the rate found. An estimate of the approximate prevalence rate likely to be found must be made and the size of the sample required can then be determined from tables. A recent WHO publication[1] deals well with the topic and is indispensable for surveys on hookworm infection or anaemia.

One-sample situations

Estimating a prevalence in a population with specified absolute precision

Required information and notation

(a) Anticipated population prevalence P
(b) Confidence level $100\,(1-\alpha)\,\%$
(c) Absolute precision required on either side
     of the prevalence (in percentage points) d

A rough estimate of anticipated prevalence P will usually suffice. If it is not possible to estimate P, a figure of 0.5 (i.e. 50% of the population is infected) should be used (as in Example 2); this is the "safest" choice for the population prevalence since the sample size required is largest when $P = 0.5$. If the anticipated prevalence is given as a range, the value closest to 0.5 should be used.

Table A3-1 presents minimum sample sizes for a confidence level of 95%.

Simple random sampling is unlikely to be the sampling method of choice in an actual field survey. If another sampling method is used, a larger sample size is likely to be needed because of the "design effect". For example, for a cluster sampling strategy the design effect might be estimated as 2. This would mean that, to obtain the same precision, twice as many individuals would have to be studied as with the simple random

---

[1] LWANGA, S. K. & LEMESHOW, S. *Sample size determination in health studies. A practical manual.* Geneva, World Health Organization, 1991.

Table A3-1. Estimating a prevalence in a population proportion with specified absolute precision

$$n = z_{1-\alpha/2}^2 P(1-P)/d^2$$

Confidence level 95%

P d	0.05	0.10	0.15	0.20	0.25	0.30	0.35	0.40	0.45
0.01	1825	3457	4898	6147	7203	8067	8740	9220	9508
0.02	456	864	1225	1537	1801	2017	2185	2305	2377
0.03	203	384	544	683	800	896	971	1024	1056
0.04	114	216	306	384	450	504	546	576	594
0.05	73	138	196	246	288	323	350	369	380
0.06	51	96	136	171	200	224	243	256	264
0.07	37	71	100	125	147	165	178	188	194
0.08	29	54	77	96	113	126	137	144	149
0.09	23	43	60	76	89	100	108	114	117
0.10	18	35	49	61	72	81	87	92	95
0.11	15	29	40	51	60	67	72	76	79
0.12	13	24	34	43	50	56	61	64	66
0.13	11	20	29	36	43	48	52	55	56
0.14	9	18	25	31	37	41	45	47	49
0.15	8	15	22	27	32	36	39	41	42
0.20	5	9	12	15	18	20	22	23	24
0.25	*	6	8	10	12	13	14	15	15

*Sample size less than 5.

sampling strategy. In Example 2, for instance, a sample size of 192 would be needed if a cluster sampling strategy were used.

Example 1

Village health workers wish to estimate the prevalence of hookworm among children under five years of age in their village. How many children should be included in the sample so that the prevalence may be estimated to within 5 percentage points of the true value with 95% confidence, if it is known that the true rate is unlikely to exceed 20%?

Solution

(*a*) Anticipated population prevalence   20%
(*b*) Confidence level   95%
(*c*) Absolute precision (15%–25%)   5 percentage points

Table A3-1 shows that for $P = 0.20$ and $d = 0.05$ a sample size of 246 would be needed.

If it is impractical, with respect to time and money, to examine 246 children, the investigators should lower their requirements of confidence.

0.50	0.55	0.60	0.65	0.70	0.75	0.80	0.85	0.90	0.95
9604	9508	9220	8740	8067	7203	6147	4898	3457	1825
2401	2377	2305	2185	2017	1801	1537	1225	864	456
1067	1056	1024	971	896	800	683	544	384	203
600	594	576	546	504	450	384	306	216	114
384	380	369	350	323	288	246	196	138	73
267	264	256	243	224	200	171	136	96	51
196	194	188	178	165	147	125	100	71	37
150	149	144	137	126	113	96	77	54	29
119	117	114	108	100	89	76	60	43	23
96	95	92	87	81	72	61	49	35	18
79	79	76	72	67	60	51	40	29	15
67	66	64	61	56	50	43	34	24	13
57	56	55	52	48	43	36	29	20	11
49	49	47	45	41	37	31	25	18	9
43	42	41	39	36	32	27	22	15	8
24	24	23	22	20	18	15	12	9	5
15	15	15	14	13	12	10	8	6	*

If there are fewer than 246 children under 5 years of age in the village, other statistical tables can be consulted for sample sizes with a lower confidence limit.

Example 2

An investigator working for a national programme of hookworm control seeks to estimate the proportion of children in the country who are receiving appropriate treatment. How many children must be studied if the resulting estimate is to fall within 10 percentage points of the true proportion with 95% confidence? (It is not possible to make any assumption regarding the treatment coverage.)

Solution

(a) Anticipated population proportion   50%
    ("safest" choice, since P is unknown)
(b) Confidence level   95%
(c) Absolute precision (40%–60%)   10 percentage points

Table A3-1 shows that for $P=0.50$ and $d=0.10$ a sample size of 96 would be required.

Hypothesis testing for a rate

Required information and notation

(a)	Test value under the null hypothesis	P_0
(b)	Anticipated value	P_a
(c)	Level of significance	$100\alpha\%$
(d)	Power of the test	$100(1-\beta)\%$
(e)	Alternative hypothesis (two-sided test)	$P_a \neq P_0$

Sometimes it is necessary to compare two rates in order to detect whether there is a significant difference between them. The probability that a test will produce a significant difference at a given significance level is called the "power" of the test. For a given test, the "power" will be dependent on the differences between the rates compared, the significance level chosen and the sample size. The following examples are for a significance level of 5% and a power of 80%. Tables are available for different combinations of power and level of significance. In determining the sample size, n, in a two-sided test, two values may be found depending on which value of P_a is used in the formula shown in Table A3–2. Since the true value of P_a is not known, the larger value of n should be taken.

Table A3-2 Hypothesis testing for a rate, two-sided test

$$n = \{z_{1-\alpha/2}\sqrt{[P_0(1-P_0)]} + z_{1-\beta}\sqrt{[P_a(1-P_a)]}\}^2/(P_0 - P_a)^2$$

Level of significance 5%, power 80%

$|P_a - P_0|$	0.05	0.10	0.15	0.20	0.25
0.01	3933	7250	10172	12701	14837
0.02	1031	1856	2582	3209	3737
0.03	478	844	1164	1440	1673
0.04	280	485	664	818	947
0.05	185	316	430	528	610
0.10	53	86	114	137	157
0.15	26	41	53	63	71
0.20	16	24	31	36	41
0.25	11	16	20	24	26
0.30	8	12	14	17	18
0.35	6	9	11	12	13
0.40	5	7	8	9	10
0.45	*	6	7	7	8
0.50	*	5	5	6	6

X is the smaller of P_0 and $(1-P_0)$.
* Sample size less than 5.

Table A3–2 is constructed so that only the larger value of n is given. Moreover, when P_0 is larger than 0.50, the complement $(1-P_0)$ should be used as the column value in this table.

Example 3

In hookworm control programmes, the six-month cure rate is estimated to be 60%. A health officer wishes to determine whether the cure rate among schoolchildren in his district was similar to the expected cure rate. What is the minimum sample size needed to determine whether an acceptable cure rate within 10 percentage points was achieved with an 80% power of detecting such a difference at the 5% level of significance?

Solution

(a) Estimated cure rate (P_0)		60%
(b) Anticipated cure rate (P_a)		$< 50\%$ or $> 70\%$
(c) Level of significance		5%
(d) Power of the test		80%
(e) Alternative hypothesis (two-sided test)		cure rate $\neq 60\%$

Table A3-2 shows that for $(1-P_0) = 0.40$ and $|P_a-P_0| = 0.10$, a sample size of 191 is required.

0.30	0.35	0.40	0.45	0.50
16580	17930	18888	19453	19626
4167	4499	4732	4868	4905
1861	2006	2107	2165	2179
1052	1132	1188	1219	1225
676	727	761	780	783
172	184	191	195	194
78	82	85	86	85
44	46	48	48	47
28	30	30	30	29
20	20	21	20	20
14	15	15	15	14
11	11	11	11	10
8	8	8	8	7
7	7	6	6	*

Example 4

In a particular district, the prevalence of hookworm in the general population was estimated to be 35%. The neighbouring district health officer wishes to know whether the prevalence in her district is similar. How many people should be examined in the neighbouring district in order to be 80% confident of detecting a difference of 5% at the 5% level of significance?

Solution

(*a*) Prevalence in first district   35%
(*b*) Anticipated prevalence in neighbouring district < 30% or > 40%
(*c*) Level of significance   5%
(*d*) Power of the test   80%
(*e*) Alternative hypothesis (two-sided test)   prevalence ≠ 35%

From Table A3-2 it can be seen that for $P_0 = 0.35$ and $|P_a - P_0| = 0.05$, a sample size of 727 is needed.

If the population is small enough, the best estimates are obtained by surveying the entire population. Usually the population is very large, and resources and time will not allow a survey of the whole population. A sample is therefore studied in order to obtain the estimates.

In practice, the population size is very much greater than the sample size, n, required to fulfil the specified precision, level of significance and power of the test. The formulae used for calculating n assume sampling from an infinite population and are approximations of the exact formulae which take into account the size of the population. These approximations are conservative, i.e. give values of n that may be larger than if the exact formulae were used. If the sample size required for an infinite population is larger than the size of the population being studied, as may be the case where a high degree of precision is demanded, then it is safe to sample one-half of the population. The real purpose of sampling is to keep n relatively low compared with the population size. Thus, if the demand for high precision calls for sampling more than two-thirds of the population, it may be advantageous to study the entire population rather than a sample.

If the population is relatively small, the sample size needed to obtain the required precision can be obtained by multiplying the sample size determined for an infinite population by a correction factor whose value is less than 1. Table A3-3 gives values for this correction factor based on the relationship between the sample size determined for an infinite population and the size of the finite population.

Table A3-3. Correction factor for sampling from a finite population

$\dfrac{\text{Sample size for infinite population}}{\text{Finite population size}} \times 100\%$	Factor by which sample size for infinite population is multiplied to obtain sample size for finite population
5	0.95
10	0.91
15	0.87
20	0.83
25	0.80
30	0.77
35	0.74
40	0.71
45	0.69
50	0.67
55	0.65
60	0.63
65	0.61
70	0.59
75	0.57
80	0.56
85	0.54
90	0.53
95	0.51
100	0.50
105	0.49
110	0.48
115	0.47
120	0.45
125	0.44
130	0.43
135	0.43
140	0.42
145	0.41
150	0.40
160	0.38
170	0.37
180	0.36
190	0.34
200	0.33

In Example 1 on page 90, it was determined that a sample of 246 children was needed in order to estimate within 5 percentage points of the true value with 95% confidence. If the total population of children under 5 years in the village was 500, the sample size would be almost 50% of the available children. From the table, the correction factor corresponding to 50% is 0.67. The sample size 246 should therefore be multiplied by 0.67, i.e. 165 children out of the 500 should be examined to obtain a precision of 5 percentage points around the anticipated rate.